IMMUNOLOGY AND IMMUNE SYSTEM DISORDERS

RHEUMATOID ARTHRITIS: PREVALENCE, RISK FACTORS AND HEALTH EFFECTS

IMMUNOLOGY AND IMMUNE SYSTEM DISORDERS

Additional books in this series can be found on Nova's website under the Series tab.

Additional E-books in this series can be found on Nova's website under the E-books tab.

IMMUNOLOGY AND IMMUNE SYSTEM DISORDERS

RHEUMATOID ARTHRITIS: PREVALENCE, RISK FACTORS AND HEALTH EFFECTS

MICHAEL H. MADSEN
EDITOR

Nova Science Publishers, Inc.
New York

For permission to use material from this book please contact us:
Telephone 631-231-7269; Fax 631-231-8175
Web Site: http://www.novapublishers.com

Additional color graphics may be available in the e-book version of this book.

Library of Congress Cataloging-in-Publication Data

Rheumatoid arthritis : prevalence, risk factors, and health effects /
editor, Michael H. Madsen.
p. ; cm.
Includes bibliographical references and index.
ISBN 978-1-61761-931-1 (hardcover)
1. Rheumatoid arthritis. I. Madsen, Michael H., 1960-
[DNLM: 1. Arthritis, Rheumatoid. WE 346]
RC933.R42874 2010
616.7'227--dc22
2010036151

Published by Nova Science Publishers, Inc. + New York

Contents

Preface

Rheumatoid arthritis (RA) is a chronic inflammatory autoimmune disease characterized by progressive joint destruction resulting from chronic synovial inflammation. It leads to various degrees of disability, and ultimately has a profound impact on the social, economic, psychological, and sexual aspects of the patient's life. This book presents current research from across the globe in the study of rheumatoid arthritis, including the relevance of genetic risk factors in rheumatoid arthritis; cervical reconstruction for cervical disorders in rheumatoid arthritis; subclinical atherosclerosis in patients with rheumatoid and psoriatic arthritis; and hand involvement and quality of life effects on patients with rheumatoid arthritis.

Chapter 1 - It is well established that, in autoimmune diseases, there is a chronic systemic inflammatory process that predominantly affects the joints. This has a significant negative impact on the quality of life of patients, and considerable socio-economic costs. In addition, in recent years a decline in life expectancy has been observed, either due to the complications of the disease itself or as a consequence of the treatments used. The most important predictors of mortality are the presence of a rheumatoid factor, the results of the Health Assessment Questionnaire (HAQ) and extra-articular manifestations. Given this increase in mortality, studies of the prognostic factors and the causes of death have been carried out, using rheumatoid arthritis (RA) and systemic lupus erythematosus (SLE) as models of autoimmune diseases.

Chapter 2 - Rheumatoid Arthritis (RA) is a chronic, inflammatory, incurable disorder of uncertain etiology, associated with significant morbidity. It is a systemic autoimmune disorder characterized by symmetric inflammation of synovial joints leading to progressive erosion of cartilage and bone. Patients require potentially lifelong treatment and there may be a substantial socio-economic impact. Generally, the onset of RA is seen in middle age (40–70 years), with a 2.5- fold higher prevalence in women than in men. Genetic polymorphisms of the major histocompatibility complex (MHC) II have been implicated in a predisposition to RA in various ethnic groups. The clinical criteria for RA has been extensively reviewed.

Joint stiffness is the cardinal clinical symptom of RA, which frequently affects the upper limb, rendering the affected limb disabled. The known pathophysiology of RA affected joint includes inflammation which produces numerous chemical mediators resulting in central sensitization causing hyperalgesia. But the nature and cause of the stiffness need to be elucidated. For this to be studied, the underlying pathophysiology and the current understanding need to be reviewed.

Chapter 3 - Rheumatoid arthritis (RA) is a chronic, inflammatory, progressive and systemic disease. Hand and wrist are the first involved parts in RA and this situation seriously affects the hand functions. Hand functions are quite important in daily living activities. Hand involvement and hand functions, are the major determinant of the course of disease and important cause of RA related disabilities. Problems in rheumatoid hand seen in different types. It is possible to classify the problems according to manifestation, anatomical parts or pathological conditions. In order to be successful in rheumatoid hand therapy it is important to understand the pathogenesis of the problem. Basically, after the pathological stages such as, tenosynovitis, tendon rupture, edema, subluxation, laxity, nodule development, contracture, functional uses of hand is limited. Early recognizing and treatment of problems in hand will increase the life quality of patient. Because lesions in RA are progressive and deformities develops during disease period. So, which methods will be helpful for doctors in diagnosis of these processes in early period? What is the position of physical examination in this methods. Besides of assessment of mentioned pathologies one by one, hand functions should be assessed globally. Many indicators been developed for this. But it is important to note that the clinic uses of these indicators are not practical and seems the differences in personal, professional and social necessities of individuals. Basically, it is very important to observe the patient continuous, to keep the deformity at minimum level and prevent them without new formations during the RA treatment. There are several types of treatment including different multidisciplinary approaches for every problem.

Chapter 4 - Rheumatoid arthritis (RA) is an autoimmune disease that affects approximately 1% of the population worldwide. RA etiology is complex, with both genetic and environmental factors influencing predisposition. Twin and family studies suggest that around 60% of heritability is due to genetic factors, being the *HLA-DRB1 locus* in he major histocompatibility complex (MHC) the main contributor. The shared epitope (SE) hypothesis pointed to a short amino acid sequence common to all *HLA-DRB1* alleles as the primary susceptibility factor associated with RA. This region has been consistently associated with RA across all populations. However, it is unclear whether the MHC *locus* predisposes to RA *per se* or owing to the development of anti-citrullinated peptide antibodies, which in turn would predispose to RA.

Different approaches have been used in the past to identify the genes associated with RA outside of the MHC. One effective approach to discover risk alleles in RA has been the candidate gene approach. This kind of studies led to the description of the tyrosine-phospatase gene *PTPN22* as a susceptibility factor for RA.

The identification of the *STAT4* polymorphism rs7574865 as a susceptibility factor for RA is an example of a combined strategy between linkage and case-control studies. Initially, Remmers *et al.* selected candidate genes from a linkage region of 52 Mb on chromosome 2q, previously defined by Amos *et al.* They performed the corresponding fine mapping, and the top associated marker, rs7574865, maped to the *STAT4* gene.

During the past 3 years, SNP genotyping technologies of high throughput have allowed investigators to efficiently screen common variation across the human genome. Genome–wide association studies (GWAS) combined this technology with large case-control collections to identify associated alleles. Several associations at *TRAF1-C5, 6q23*, *TNFAIP3* or *REL loci* have been independently described by this kind of analysis.

Although much of the recent excitement in the field has resulted from the utilization of GWAS to search for genes outside the MHC, it is important to remember some things.

Firstly, the single most important contribution to genetic risk for RA clearly resides within the MHC. Secondly, validated non-MHC RA risk alleles only explain 5% of the genetic weight of disease, and finally, GWAS had been performed at European ancestry cohorts so it will be of particular interest to conduct these GWAS in collections of non-European ancestry.

In summary, approximately half of the genetic susceptibility to RA remains to be explained at present.

Chapter 5 - To reconstruct highly destructed unstable rheumatoid arthritis (RA) cervical lesions, the authors have been using C1/2 transarticular and cervical pedicle screw fixations. Pedicle screw fixation and C1/2 transarticular screw fixation are biomechanically superior to other fixation techniques for RA patients. However, due to severe spinal deformity and small anatomical size of the vertebra, including the lateral mass and pedicle, in the most RA cervical lesions, these screw fixation procedures are technically demanding and pose the potential risk of neurovascular injuries. The purpose of this study was to evaluate the long-term results of cervical reconstruction for the deformed, fragile, and small RA spine lesions using computer-assisted image-guidance systems. A frameless, stereotactic image-guidance system that is CT-based, and optoelectronic was used for correct screw placement. A total of 20 patients (14 females, 6 males) with cervical disorders due to RA were surgically treated using the image-guidance system.

Postoperative computerized tomography was used to determine the accuracy of the screw placement. Neural and vascular complications associated with screw insertion and postoperative neural recovery were evaluated. Postoperative radiological evaluations revealed that only 1 (2.5%; C4) of 40 screws inserted into the cervical pedicle had perforated more than 50% of the screw diameter (critical breach). However, no neurovascular complications were observed. According to Ranawat's classification, 8 patients remained the same, 11 patients showed improvement, and 1 patient showed deterioration. Instrumentation failure, loss of reduction, or nonunion was not observed at the final follow-up (average 49 months; range 24–108 months). In this study, the authors demonstrated that image-guidance systems could be applied safely to the cervical lesions caused by RA. Image-guidance systems are useful tools in preoperative planning and in transarticular or transpedicular screw placement in the cervical spine of RA patients.

Chapter 6 - Rheumatoid arthritis (RA) is a chronic inflammatory autoimmune disease characterized by progressive joint destruction resulting from chronic synovial inflammation. It leads to various degrees of disability, and ultimately has a profound impact on the social, economic, psychological, and sexual aspects of the patient's life. The percentage of arthritic patients who experience sexual problems ranged in various studies from 31 to 76%. The reasons for disturbing sexual functioning are multifactorial and comprise disease-related factors as well as therapy. It can occur before, during and after sexual activities, and can affect sexual health in different perspectives.

Sexuality is a complex aspect of the human being's life and is more than of only the sexual act. Normal sexual functioning consists of sexual activity with transition through the phases from arousal to relaxation with no problems, and with a feeling of pleasure, fulfillment and satisfaction. Rheumatic diseases may affect all aspects of life including sexual functioning.

The treatment of sexual dysfunction will depend on the specific patient's symptoms, however, there are some general recommendations including: exploring different positions, using analgesics drug, heat and muscle relaxants before sexual activity and exploring alternative methods of sexual expression.

There are not enough studies comparing sexual functioning between RA patients and healthy controls. However, there is a tendency to find more sexual functioning problems in patients with RA. These patients could experience sexual disability and diminish sexual drive, with pain and depression being the most common symptoms. This chapter is about the impact of RA on sexual functioning.

Chapter 7 - Activated human T cells produce receptor activator NF-κB ligand (RANKL), interleukin-17 (IL-17), and interferon-γ (IFN-γ). All regulate human osteoclastogenesis; RANKL and IL-17 potently induce osteoclastogenesis, while IFN-γ directly inhibits it in vitro. However, we have demonstrated that IFN-γ-producing T cells induce human osteoclastogenesis from monocytes through the expression of RANKL. Strongly supporting our findings, it has been reported that peripheral blood T cells from patients with early rheumatoid arthritis (RA) promote osteoclastogenesis in autologus monocytes through the expression of RANKL, although the T cells express IFN-γ. In addition, it has been reported that IFN-γ has indirect pro-osteoclastogenic properties in vivo; IFN-γ induces bone resorption in three mouse models of osteoporosis under conditions of estrogen deficiency, infection, and inflammation. On the other hand, the expression or function of some cytokines shows differences between humans and mice in bone cell biology. In the current article, we review recent findings on the role of T cells in human osteoclastogenesis and bone destruction of rheumatoid arthritis (RA), including the effects of dexamethasone and tacrolimus on the function of T cells.

Chapter 8 - Accelerated development of atherosclerosis has been observed in patients with rheumatic diseases such as rheumatoid arthritis (RA) and psoriatic arthritis (PsA). It may be related to the inflammatory overload accompanied to the combination of an excessive production of reactive oxygen species with an impaired antioxidant defence capacity, leading to oxidative stress that may facilitate the development and progression of atherosclerosis. Compared with the general population, patients with RA die prematurely, mainly because of cardiovascular diseases but the mechanism by which premature atherosclerosis develops in RA is unknown. Recent data have demonstrated the prevalence of atherosclerosis also in patients with PsA, a chronic inflammatory autoimmune disease characterized by inflammatory arthritis and skin psoriasis. PsA shares some phenotypic characteristics with RA, even though the synovial inflammation of PsA is characterized by less macrophage infiltration and increased vascularity in comparison to RA inflammation. The increased cardiovascular risk in PsA and RA suggests the need to treat the inflammatory process and to monitor traditional atherosclerotic risk factors in these pathologies.

The aim of our study was to evaluate whether increased oxidative stress may be associated to the presence of subclinical atherosclerosis in patients with RA and in patients with PsA. For this purpose we determined the levels of oxidized low density lipoproteins (ox-LDL) and of nitric oxide (NO) in the sera obtained from 19 patients with RA, 20 with PsA and 20 sex- and age-matched healthy controls. Patients with RA fulfilled the American College of Rheumatology criteria, and patients with PsA fulfilled the CASPAR criteria. In all patients we evaluated the activity and duration of the disease and classical risk factors for atherosclerosis. Our results showed higher levels of ox-LDL and lower levels of NO in sera from patients with RA and PsA than in sera from healthy controls. Notably, higher serum levels of ox-LDL were observed in patients with an intima-media thickness (IMT) >1 than in those with an IMT ≤ 1, and higher serum levels of NO in patients with an IMT ≤ 1 than in those with an IMT >1, in patients with RA and PsA. Our data suggest that monitoring circulating levels of ox-LDL and NO in patients with RA and PsA could give information on the development of atherosclerotic disease and therefore could be useful to the clinical management of patients.

In: Rheumatoid Arthritis: Prevalence, Risk…
Editor: Michael H. Madsen
ISBN: 978-1-61761-931-1

Chapter 1

Pathogenesis Mechanism and Cardiovascular Risk Factors for Arteriosclerosis in Rheumatoid Arthritis: The Importance and Implications of Early Diagnosis

Alberto López de Guzmán[1], Juan de Dios García Díaz[1], María Isabel Díez-Pérez de la Vacas[2], Eduardo Cuende Quintana[3], Ana Sánchez Atrio[3] and Iliana Sivera Monzó[4]

[a]Internal medicine, [b]Radiology, [c]Rheumatology and [d]Biochemistry Services, Príncipe de Asturias University Hospital., University of Alcalá., Alcalá de Henares. Madrid

1. The Impact of Cardiovascular Disease on Morbimortality in Rheumatoid Arthritis

It is well established that, in autoimmune diseases, there is a chronic systemic inflammatory process that predominantly affects the joints. This has a significant negative impact on the quality of life of patients, and considerable socio-economic costs.[1] In addition, in recent years a decline in life expectancy has been observed,[2,3] either due to the complications of the disease itself or as a consequence of the treatments used. The most important predictors of mortality are the presence of a rheumatoid factor, the results of the Health Assessment Questionnaire (HAQ) and extra-articular manifestations. Given this increase in mortality, studies of the prognostic factors and the causes of death have been carried out, using rheumatoid arthritis (RA) and systemic lupus erythematosus (SLE) as models of autoimmune diseases.

The majority of studies of RA describe a high rate of mortality in comparison with the general population or control groups. Fundamentally they consisted of prospective cohort studies carried out with patients in hospitals, though these were not necessarily in-patients, with a follow-up period that varied between 3 and 35 years. A minority of studies are descriptive studies of participant and control groups. The measure most often used to measure the mortality of patients with RA is the standardised mortality rate (SMR). This is described as the relationship between observed mortality and expected mortality.[4]

Cardiovascular disease (CD) is described as the principal cause of death in patients with RA in the majority of the studies.[5] The influence of CD is so significant in morbimortality in people with RA that it is estimated that it reduces life expectancy of these patients by some 3-18 years compared to the general population. Consequently, the life expectancy of people with RA has been said to be similar to that of people suffering from stage IV Hodgkin's disease or three-vessel coronary heart disease[6-8]. This increase in mortality as a result of CD in people with RA occurs in both men and women.[9] Within the causes of death due to CD, ischemic heart disease has been described as the most frequent, followed by cerebrovascular disease. Wolfe et al[10] in a study of 3,501 patients found that the principal cause of death in patients with RA was CD with an SMR of 2.26. Wallberg-Jonsson[11] also found that the most frequent cause of mortality was CD in 53% of cases, and of these the most frequent cause was ischemic heart disease with an SMR of 3.

This concern regarding the influence of CD on the mortality of patients with RA has continued during the first years of the 21st century. Of particular importance is a study completed in Rochester (Minnesota) in 2005.[12] The study involved a cohort of 603 patients with RA living in Rochester of whom 73% were women, with an average age of 58. They were followed up for 15 years. It was observed that, in 176 of the 354 patients who died, the cause of death was CD. This principally involved patients with systemic inflammation (a high erythrocyte sedimentation rate) and was statistically significant and independent of traditional risk factors. In contrast to the increase that occurred in the past in mortality secondary to CD in people with RA, in recent years a reduction in mortality has been observed. For example, in a study carried out with a cohort of 3,862 patients[13] with RA followed up for 15 years, it was found that mortality as a result of ischemic heart disease gradually fell over the years, coinciding with the use of disease modifying medication, such as methotrexate.

In patients with SLE, a systemic chronic inflammatory disease, the importance of CD as a cause of mortality has also been studied.[14] Urowitz et al[15] were the first to indicate the importance of CD in the long-term progress of patients with SLE. A bimodal pattern of mortality was described in which earlier deaths were due to the activity of disease or infections, whereas later deaths (9 years after diagnosis) were due to ischemic heart disease. In the 1980s, mortality attributable to CD was around 20%, depending on the number of patients in the series, but recently mortality rates of 75% attributable to CD have been found.[16,17]

In short, it is currently considered that RA as a chronic systemic inflammatory disease not only influences the quality of life of the patients that suffer from it but is also associated with a reduction in life expectancy. In recent years it has been observed that this increase in mortality is due to CD, as it is in the general population, but that those with this disease have a higher SMR. Both sexes are affected by this. Within CD and independent of traditional risk factors, ischemic heart disease is particularly significant, followed by cerebrovascular disease. Therefore, in RA *accelerated arteriosclerosis* develops, which can be explained by the systemic inflammatory process itself [18] as can be seen in the following sections, and RA can be considered as a vascular risk factor (see Figure 1).

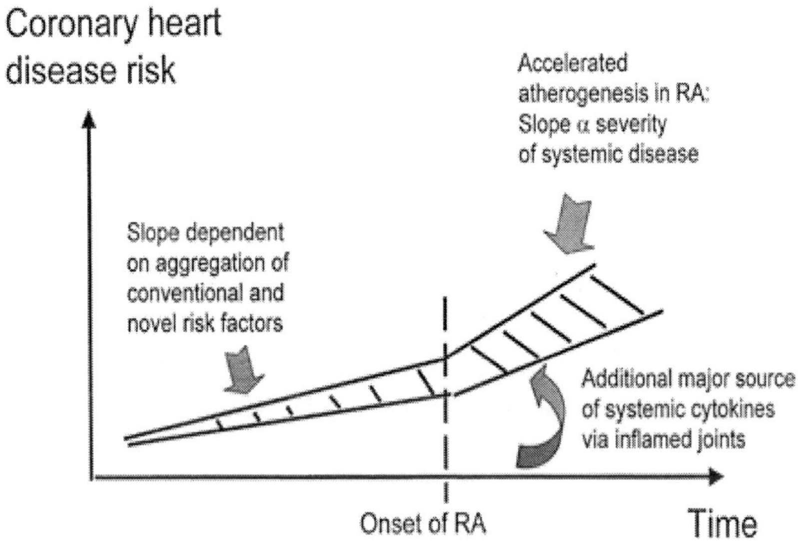

Figure 1. Before the diagnosis of RA, the classic vascular risk factors are greater influences on CD, but after the diagnosis of the disease it is systemic inflammation that explains the accelerated arteriosclerosis. **Reference film 35*

2. The Pathogenesis of Accelerated Arteriosclerosis in RA

The cause of the high and premature death rates in patients with RA is not precisely known. It is currently thought that accelerated arteriosclerosis influences various mechanisms, among which in particular are: traditional vascular risk factors; new vascular risk factors; the dual effect of the medication used to treat the disease, as discussed below, and the inflammatory phenomenon (see Figure 2).

This last mechanism is currently considered to be the best explanation for accelerated arteriosclerosis, based on the current theory that the atheromatous plaque is basically an inflammatory process[19-22] involving cellular and molecular elements present in the physiopathy of RA, as explained below. It can be considered that the arterial condition in the autoimmune disease is due to vasculitis rather than early arteriosclerosis. This has also been studied, although, as post-mortem examination and anatomopathological studies of the arteries of patients who die from CD is needed, this is more difficult to carry out. The pathological findings of different studies include periocarditis, myocarditis, angitis, granulomatous lesions and amyloid deposits, but with a much lower frequency than expected, not explaining death due to cardiovascular causes. For example, Van Albada-Kuipers et al,[23]in a series of 173 autopsies, found 17 cases of systemic vasculitis, of which only 4 had coronary involvement, and Karten[24]carried out 102 autopsies, finding 6 cases of systemic vasculitis and one case of coronary vasculitis.

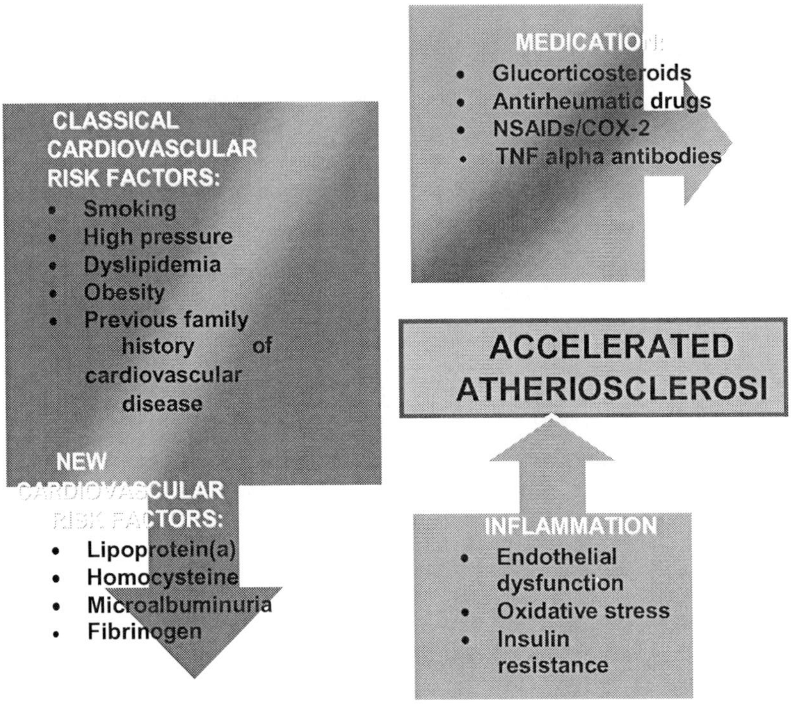

Figure 2. Accelerated arteriosclerosis mechanisms in rheumatoid arthritis

On the other hand, it has been postulated that a hereditary factor can influence accelerated arteriosclerosis, similar to that occurring in the general population. For example, in a study carried out recently in Sweden,[25] 10,805 patients with RA aged between 16 and 67 were followed up over 10 years. It was observed that having a family history of CD was associated with an increase of more than 70% in death from CD compared to those who did not have such a history. This represents an SMR for ischemic heart disease of 2.9%.

Finally, this excessively high mortality rate justifies the study of risk factors and the use of diagnostic methods in order to detect patients with a greater risk of the disease as early as possible, and beginning more aggressive therapies to reduce the intrinsic inflammatory activity of the disease itself. Consequently, numerous studies have been carried out over the last decade with patients with SLE and RA, using diagnostic methods for sub-clinical arteriosclerosis. These methods particularly include measuring the intima-media thickness (IMT) by carotid ultrasound in the diagnosis of sub-clinical cerebrovascular disease, using CT scans to quantify coronary calcium in the study of sub-clinical coronary arteriopathy and the ankle-brachial index (ABI) for the study of peripheral arteriopathy. These diagnostic methods and their application to RA are described in the following section.

2.1. Inflammatory Mechanisms in the Formation of Atheromatous Plaques

Arteriosclerotic disease is characterised by the thickening and hardening of arterial walls due to the accumulation of lipid material, fibrous tissue and calcium deposits in the sub-endothelial space, resulting in the reduction of the arterial lumen with the consequent development of ischemic events. Arteriosclerosis is therefore a unique pathological entity that affects different arterial areas of the body.

Currently it has been clearly demonstrated that the risk of an ischemic event occurring depends fundamentally on the composition of the arteriosclerotic lesions and not so much on the degree of arterial stenosis as was classically believed. Different theories have therefore been postulated regarding the origin and development of atheromatous plaque, the most accepted theories being the lipid theory and thrombogenic theory. Currently, the predominant theory is the multi-factoral theory that incorporates all the above theories, and which is based on the idea that the formation of atheromatous plaque is principally an inflammatory phenomenon. The phases of this process are described below. These are then are related to the pro-atherogenic process present in autoimmune diseases, using RA as a model. The phases are: endothelia dysfunction, the accumulation and oxidation of lipoproteins, the recruitment of leukocytes, the formation of foam cells, the synthesis of the components of the extra-cellular matrix and apoptosis.

The pillar on which the origin of the arteriosclerotic lesion is based is endothelial dysfunction. The endothelium is currently considered to be the source and target for a series of vaso-active agents, in such a way that it has an endocrine and paracrine action, not only on the endothelium but also on the neighbouring smooth muscle cells. These actions are carried out by means of nitric oxide (NO) after the activation of the nitric oxide synthase (eNO), with a predominantly protective effect in relation to arteriosclerosis, as it inhibits plaque aggregation, LDL oxidation, expression of adhesion molecules, etc. Furthermore, it maintains a balance between the pro and anti-arteriogenic biochemical processes.

Endothelial Dysfunction

1. Endothelial dysfunction induces a decrease in the synthesis of the NO, with the consequent reduction in its beneficial activities, resulting in a pro-arteriosclerotic situation. This endothelial dysfunction is determined by the presence of vascular risk factors such as hyperlipidemia, tobacco, diabetes, free radicals, etc. However, another element fostering this alteration in endothelial functionality is the presence of the share rate, resulting from the speed of blood flow and the vascular radius. Thus, arterial areas with a low share rate (areas of curvature or points of arterial bifurcation) have a greater propensity to develop arteriosclerotic lesions.[26, 27]
2. This allows a greater permeability of the endothelium to plasma proteins, principally low density lipoproteins (LDL) that become the principal protagonists of the inflammatory process. The next stage is therefore the accumulation, modification and oxidation of the LDLs. These accumulate in the innermost layer of the artery due both to the greater endothelial permeability and their interaction with components of the extra-cellular matrix through the apoB, which facilitates their presence in the arterial wall[28]. Once they have entered the sub-endothelial space, the LDLs are

very susceptible to being transformed through lipolysis, aggregation and oxidation by free radicals, as they cannot be in contact with anti-oxidant agents (see Figure 3).

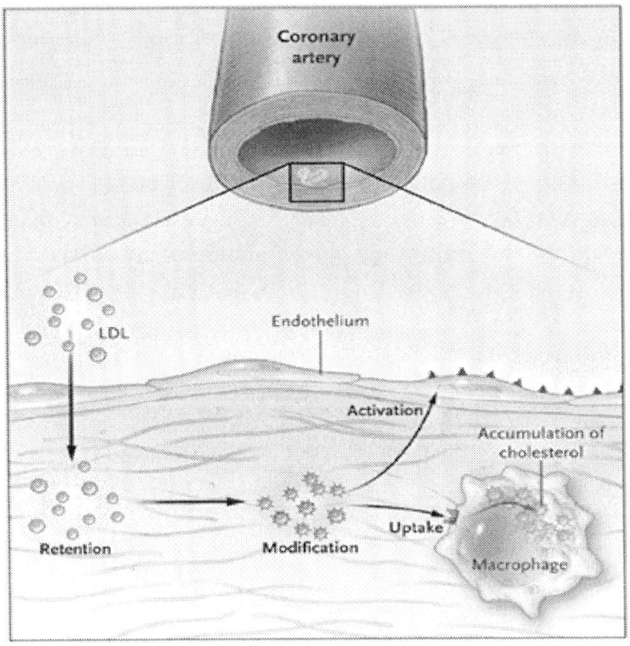

Figure 3. The effects of modified LDL * Reference film 20

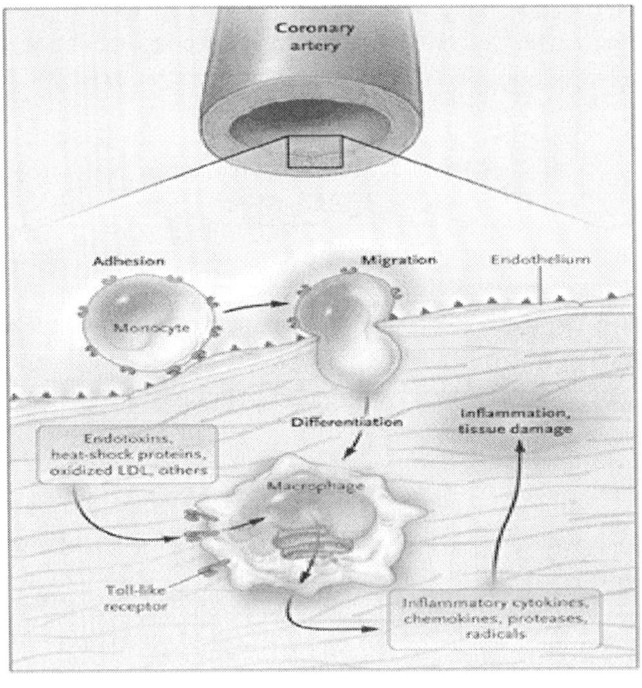

Figure 4. Adhesion and internalisation of macrophages. The. importance of their transformation into foam cells

This transformation of the LDLs is an inflammatory stimulus that is very significant for the endothelium. Its activation leads to the expression of some adhesive proteins of the selectin superfamily (L-selectin and P-selectin) which begins the recruitment of leukocytes. These proteins combine with the carbohydrates from the surface of the leukocytes and stimulate the migration of monocytes from the bloodstream towards the endothelial surface, where they adhere. After the expression of selectins, the expression of another type of adhesive proteins occurs. These are the ELAMs (endothelial-leukocyte adhesion molecules; ICAM-1 and VCAM-1). These facilitate the migration of the monocyte-lymphocytes adhering to the endothelial wall (Figure 4).

After their internalisation, the monocytes/macrophages on the wall are transformed into foamy macrophages, when their lipid content increases after phagocytising the oxidised LDL accumulated in the arterial wall. They represent the most important cellular component of fatty streaks (see Figure 6) [29,30]. The internalisation of the oxidised LDL in the macrophages is carried out by means of three types of receptors. One is the classic LDL receptor[30] which can be regulated by intracellular cholesterol values. Other receptors are the scavengers that internalise the lipid material by a mechanism that cannot be regulated. These mechanisms that cannot be regulated are characterised by the fact that, until such time as the cells are in a medium rich in lipid material, they will continue independently internalising the intracellular lipid content. Finally, another receptor that is fundamental to the inflammatory process is the toll-like receptor (also present in dendritic, mast and endothelial cells). It is characterised by the way it begins a cascade of pro-inflammatory signals such as cytokines, proteases and free radicals (see Figure 4).

These cytokines stimulate the proliferation of smooth muscle cells and the production of the extra-cellular matrix (see Figure 8). The smooth muscle cells from the activated tunica media emigrate towards the tunica intima, undergoing a change in their phenotype. This occurs in such a way that they cease to have a vasoconstrictive function and present a static function, consistent with the synthesis of the components of the extra-cellular matrix (collagen, elastin). This leads to the enlargement of the intima layer, reducing the arterial lumen. In this way, cytokines such as interleukin 1 (IL-1) and the TNF α freed by the macrophages, foster the local production of growth factors, such as the plaque growth factor and the fibroblast growth factor.

In addition to the macrophage in the arteriosclerotic lesion, the T lymphocytes, mostly CD4+Th1 lymphocytes, are also present, recognising the amphigens (principally oxidised LDL) presented, by means of type 2 (HLA II) histocompatibility molecules, principally by macrophages (see Figure 5). Subsequently a type Th1 pro-inflammatory response is initiated (retarded hypersensitivity) through the liberation of cytokines, principally interferon γ (IFNγ). This inhibits the proliferation of smooth muscle and the synthesis of the interstitial forms of collagen. However, it largely promotes the increase in the synthesis of other cytokines such as TNFα and IL-1,[31] acting synergetically (see Figure 6) and perpetuating the inflammatory process. These three cytokines stimulate the production of interleukin 6 (IL6) in the arterial lesion, in the same way as occurs in other tissues, such as the adipose tissue. IL-6 stimulates the production of acute phase reactants at a hepatic level, such as reactive C protein (RCP) or serum amyloid A (SAA) and fibrinogen. As explained below, these acute phase reactants are going to be very useful in evaluating the degree of inflammation in RA, even in its quiescent phases.

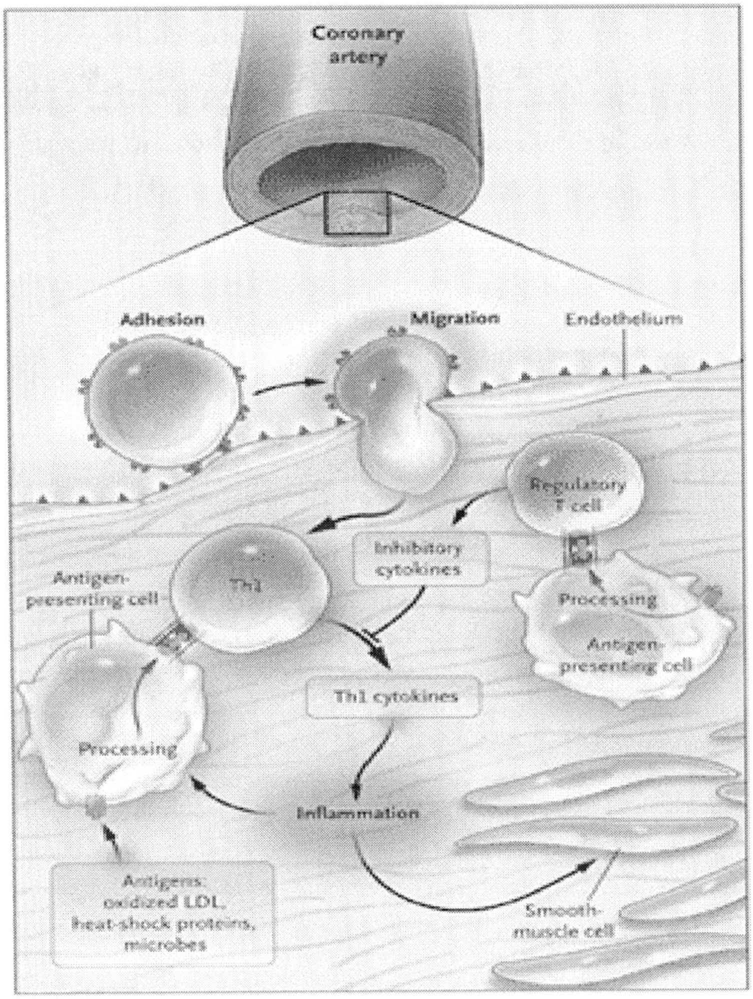

Figure 5. Activation of the T lymphocytes * *Reference film 20*

As already discussed above, there are mechanisms that cannot be regulated through which the monocytes/macrophages internalise the modified lipoproteins, independently of the intracellular lipid content. The impossibility of regulating this internalisation means that there is an excessive accumulation that can lead to cell death or apoptosis.[32] It has been postulated, therefore, that pro-inflammatory agents can trigger apoptosis of the endothelial cells, thereby setting off biochemical and molecular processes that lead to the formation of arteriosclerotic lesions.[33,34]

After apoptosis of the macrophages, the vulnerability of the arteriosclerotic lesion increases and leads to the release of its content into tissue factor. When these lesions rich in tissue factor break up and come into contact with the circulating blood, this can lead to the acute formation of a very large thrombosis, which will very probably lead to an ischemic process. The apoptosis can therefore be considered as a connecting link between the inflammation and the thrombotic complications of arteriosclerosis.

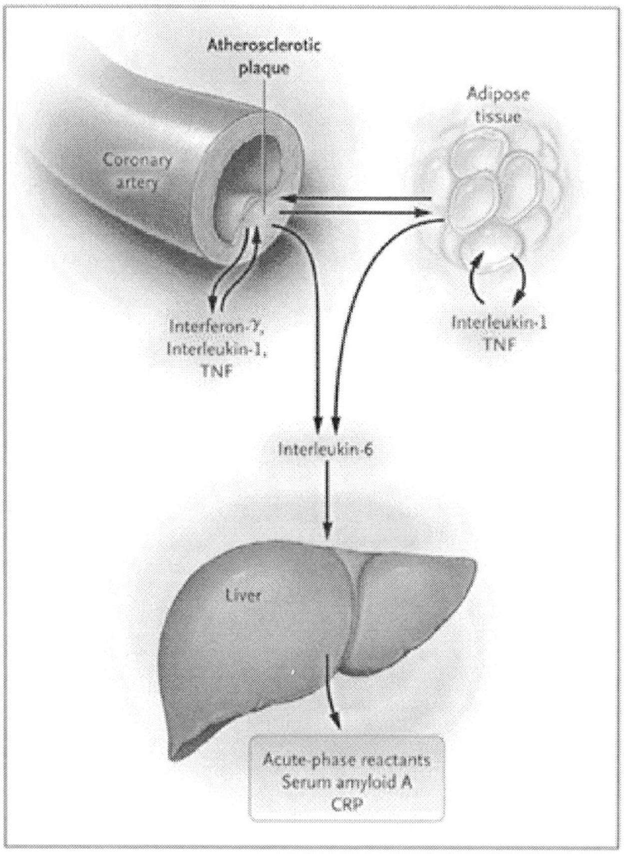

Figure 6. Synergetic action of the cytokines * *Reference film 20*

2.2. The Metabolic and Vascular Effects of Systemic Inflammation in RA

In autoimmune disease, principally in SLE and RA, the most important pro-atherogenic mechanism is chronic inflammation, which is present even in the quiescent phases of the disease i.e. a continuous inflammatory stimulus is produced.

In RA the inflammatory process is developed initially at joint level, specifically at a synovial level. From here, the cytokines are freed into the systemic circulation where they act on various tissues, principally at an adipose tissue, liver, muscle and endothelial level. Consequently, cytokines such as TNFα, IL1 and IL6 that are usually found at high levels in plasma during inflammatory processes, are also found in the synovial fluid.[35] The action of these cytokines on the different tissues induces pro-atherogenic changes, giving rise to insulin resistance, dyslipidemia, pro-thrombotic effects, oxidative stress and endothelial dysfunction (see Figure 7).

The continuous inflammatory stimulus in RA is particularly important as it is maintained even in the quiescent phases of the disease (see Figure 8). As discussed above, the degree of inflammation can be measured on the basis of the CRP levels and specifically the ultra-sensitive CRP.[36-38] CRP is a member of the pentraxin family of proteins,[39] the physiological role of which is not yet well established. It is currently is considered that their pro-inflammatory action predominates. This primarily activates the complement system and endothelial cells to express adhesion molecules.[40] Because of this, its quantification is routinely used in clinical practice for detecting and monitoring acute phase conditions.

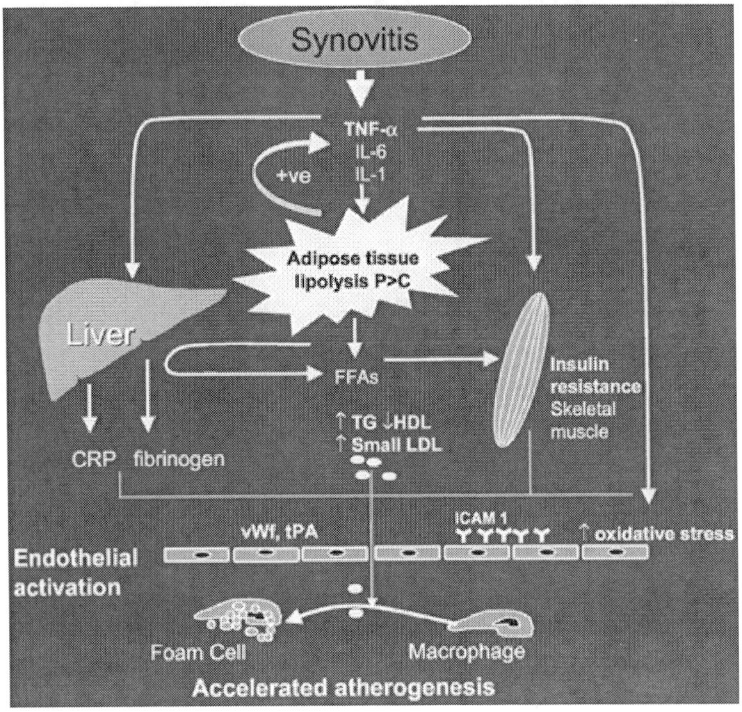

Figure 7. Systematic release of cytokines from the joint. These induce pro-atherogenic actions in various tissues. * *Reference film 35*

The development of ultra-sensitive methods for determining the CRP has made it possible to establish two ranges of values: above 10mg/l, detectable routinely, and below 10mg/l (pathological from 3mg/l), measurable by new ultra-sensitive methods. The variations in the concentration of CRP in this ultra-sensitive range are those that have been attributed to the situation known as chronic or low-intensity inflammation. This, in turn, has been identified as a powerful marker of arteriosclerotic disease.[41-43] This assertion is based on recent studies that demonstrate an association between endothelial dysfunction and low-grade inflammation, demonstrating that the level of CRP concentration correlated with a reduction in the production of NO[44].

High levels of CRP have been described in RA, probably through the activation of components of the complement system.[45] As discussed above, the CRP is synthesised at a hepatic level, in the same way as the SAA. It is also considered to be an acute phase reactant[46] and is detected in macrophages, endothelial cells and smooth muscle cells in the atheromatous plaques of these patients[47] .

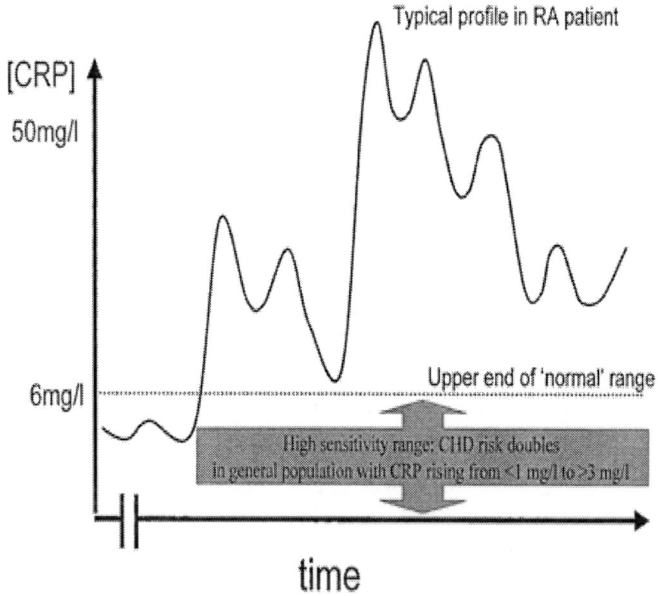

Figure 8. Inflammatory stimulus maintained in RA, even in quiescent phases-* *Reference film 35*

In the following sections current knowledge regarding the presence in RA of the different elements of the inflammatory process, leading to the development of atheromatous plaques described above, is discussed, paying particular attention to pro-athrogenic conditions. Firstly, reference is made to endothelial dysfunction in RA. This is followed by a discussion of the importance of CD4+/CD28null Th1 lymphocytes as cells of the immune system, present both in the atheromatous plaques of patients with unstable angina as in those with RA,[48] and in the haemostatic changes that occur in RA.

2.2.1. Endothelial Dysfunction In RA

The cytokines released from the joint, act on the different tissues, causing pro-atherogenic changes, as already described. One of these target tissues is endothelium. Endothelial dysfunction is the first inflammatory step, and in RA it is produced both through the pro-atherogenic lipid profile and through the reduction in NO synthesis. Various lines of research indicate the importance of NO in the inflammatory pathogenesis in RA.[49,50] It has been observed that the macrophages of the arterial lesion in RA can be activated to express an inferred form of the NO synthesising enzyme (iNO) which is characterised by its ability to produce large cytotoxic quantities of NO radicals.[51,52] Furthermore, the NO acts as a mediator in the apoptosis of the articular inflammatory process in RA [53] and as an important regulator of the Th1/Th2 balance in autoimmune diseases.[54] Finally, genetic polymorphism of eNO has been studied. This is not involved in susceptibility to RA in the general population, which implies that genes, other than eNO ones can be responsible for the expression of cytokines and other pro-inflammatory elements that are involved in susceptibility to the disease. By contrast, in a recent study in this country[55], significant differences have been found in the genetic polymorphism of patients with RA compared to the control group. It is therefore important to take account of the role this genetic polymorphism can play in the pathology of RA.

Another endothelial dysfunction mechanism in RA derives from the action of TNFα on the endothelium itself. In addition to inducing a pro-atherogenic lipid environment and fostering oxidative stress,[56] the TNFα also blocks the activation of the eNO, interfering in the phosphorylation of the protein kinase Akt [57]. It also acts on the eNOmRNA[58] degrading it and thereby impeding the synthesis of eNO. Another manifestation of the presence of endothelial dysfunction in RA is the elevation of the serum levels of adhesion molecules, such as ICAM and selectins, as inflammatory markers.[59,60]

Endothelial dysfunction in the RA has not only been studied at a molecular level but also at a morphological level. The study of the endothelial function is carried out by means of ultrasound study of the brachial artery, evaluating changes in calibre of the vein with two types of stimulus (see Figure 9). The first stimulus consists of an increase in post-ischemic flow induced by a tourniquet, giving rise to the release of endothelium dependent endogenous NO and causing vasodilation in physiological conditions. The second is the administration of sublingual nitroglycerine as an exogenous donor of NO producing a vasodilation independent of the endothelium and reflecting the functioning of the arterial smooth muscle.[61] It has been observed that patients with slow-developing RA and without known CD have lower endothelium-dependent vasodilation than the general population, independently of the severity of the radiological articular involvement.[62] This has also been observed in young patients with low-severity RA[63] .

Finally, the quantity of endothelial progenitor cells (EPCs) in peripheral blood in RA has been quantified, as this correlates inversely with vascular risk. It was observed that RA is related to a depletion of EPCs in peripheral blood, and this could be one of the factors contributing to high cardiovascular risk[64]

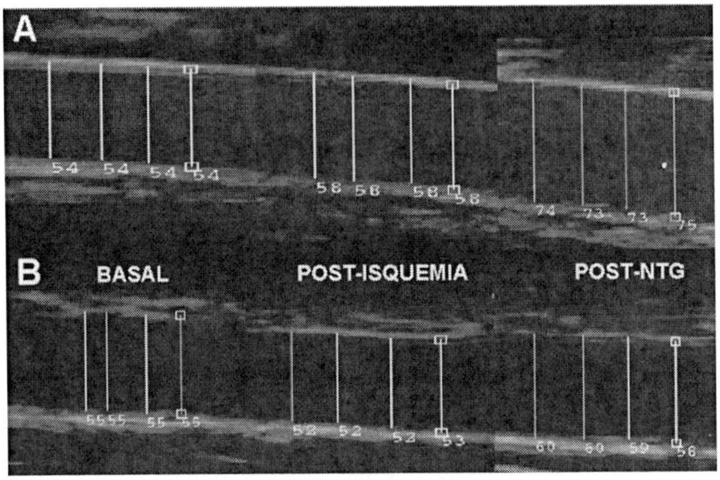

Figure 9. Evaluation of the endothelial function of the brachial artery by ultrasound * *Reference film 61*

2.2.2. CD4+/CD28null Lymphocytes

Several studies have demonstrated the presence of the CD4+/CD28null lymphocyte as the predominant cell in the inflammatory process that takes place in RA and in arteriosclerotic disease. Even so, this type of lymphocyte is not very common in the healthy population (0.1-

2.5% of the whole T lymphocyte pool)[65]. On the other hand, it has a significant presence in unstable angina,[48] multiple sclerosis, Wegener's granulomatosis, and in RA with significant extra-articular manifestations.[66-70] The clonal expansion of this lymphocyte is determined genetically, principally by blocking transcription, which also takes place before a stimulus maintained by the TNF α.[71]

The CD4+/CD28null lymphocyte participates in a delayed hypersensitivity immune response and is activated after the presentation of the antigen, principally by the HLA II antigen (see Figure 8). The fact that they do not present CD28 (a lymphocyte surface receptor that transmits co-stimulation signals after interacting with antigen-presenting cell receptors) on their surface, means that this lymphocyte has certain particular characteristics. It does not require CD28 for its activation, nor does it express another receptor with the co-stimulating function of CD80. It is not able to activate B lymphocytes. It has important cytotoxic activity and releases high levels of IFN-gamma and IL-2, even in the absence of an inflammatory stimulus.[72,73] In addition, it presents resistance to apoptosis through a mechanism that is not clear, probably through the elevated expression of anti-apoptotic Bcl-2 protein.[74]

Its cytotoxic activity is substantial despite being CD4+.[75] This peculiarity has been demonstrated through observing perforin-like proteins in lymphocytes of this type in peripheral blood and in synovial fluid. Furthermore, it expresses receptors similar to those that are present in natural killer cells (NK) such as homodimer CD8 on its surface, which explains its ability to infiltrate different tissues, amongst them the endothelium.[75,76] The role of these cells in RA is therefore based principally on their cytotoxic capacity. This can contribute to the extra-articular manifestations of the disease and the degree of articular inflammatory activity[76].

2.2.3. Haemostasis

In recent years there has been sufficient evidence of the pro-coagulant state that predominates in RA. The elevation of the fibrinogen level, the von Willebrand factor, D-dimer and tissue plasminogen activator antigen have all been demonstrated in patients with RA, even in those that are well controlled (measured by CRP levels).[77] It also contributes thrombocytosis to this pro-coagulation state in RA.[78]

It is important to highlight the fact that many of these parameters are clearly associated with the degree of inflammatory response. The mechanisms through which this pro-coagulant environment is established are not well known, but it has been observed that the TNF α induces the expression of tissue factor in monocytes and endothelium, triggering the coagulation cascade. In addition, the IL-6 increases levels of fibrinogen, which is currently considered to be an acute phase reactant[79] .

2.3. Classic Vascular Risk Factors

2.3.1. Arterial Hypertension (AHT)

The relationship between the presence of AHT and the elevation of inflammatory markers in healthy patients is well established. For example, in a study involving 508 healthy men[80] an association between the increase in arterial pressure and the elevation of the plasma of two inflammatory markers - ICAM-1 and IL-6 - was observed, in such a way that an increase in the systolic arterial pressure and average arterial pressure was associated with a significant increase in ICAM-1. In addition, all the measures of arterial pressure, including diastolic, correlate with high levels of IL-6.

These findings suggest that the continuous inflammatory process involves an increase in arterial pressure, thereby contributing to accelerated arteriosclerosis. This concept has been analysed in RA, with various studies observing an increase in arterial pressure in comparison with the general population. This has been observed in diastolic arterial pressure,[81] systolic arterial pressure and average pressure[82] .

2.3.2. Smoking

Several studies have been carried out to evaluate the relationship between smoking and arteriosclerosis in RA. Coronary heart disease in RA influenced by tobacco could be explained if it were shown that smoking was more prevalent in patients with RA than in the general population or if this were also a risk factor for the development of RA.

The majority of these studies[83-91] have not established a significant relationship. It has not been shown that the risk of CD is greater in patients with RA who smoke than in smokers who do not have RA. By contrast, RA and smoking are associated with factors that represent a greater activity of the disease, such as the presence of rheumatoid factor (RA seropositive), the presence of radiological erosions and rheumatoid nodules.[92,93]

2.3.3. Obesity

Obesity is a risk factor for CD and increases mortality in the general population, so it could potentially contribute to a greater incidence of complications deriving from arteriosclerosis in RA. This concept cannot be applied to RA, as it is a disease characterised by the loss of body mass, known as rheumatoid cachexia. In a recent retrospective study,[12] in which the relationship between the body mass index (BMI) and cardiovascular mortality in patients with RA was evaluated, it was observed that a BMI of <20kg/m2 is a predictor of increased cardiovascular mortality in these patients.

2.3.4. Dyslipidemia

As discussed above, RA presents a clear, pro-atherogenic lipid profile (table 2) that contributes to endothelial dysfunction, increasing the cardiovascular risk in these patients. The mechanisms associated with this lipid profile are the result of the action of cytokines (see Figure 10) on the adipose tissue, producing an increase in fatty acids. At hepatic level, they produce an increase in the levels of triglycerides, and in the endothelium they reduce lipoprotein lipase activity, which is the principal catabolic enzyme of triglycerides[55,56]. Other mechanisms promoting dyslipidemia are the action of medication administered for the treatment of RA and the importance of lipoprotein as a new vascular risk factor. Both are discussed below.

This has two consequences: an increase in fatty acids, which constitutes the physiopathological basis for insulin resistance, as described below, and an increase in triglycerides that lead, through neutral lipid exchange, to a reduction of HDL cholesterol and the synthesis of small, dense LDL cholesterol particles. (They are more atherogenic because they can penetrate the endothelium more easily, adhere better to the wall proteoglycans and are easier to modify through oxidation).

It is important to highlight the importance of the reduction in HDL, as it is currently considered to be the principal protector against an excessive accumulation of lipid material due to the reverse transportation of cholesterol. The mechanism whereby lipids enter the arterial wall is directly related to LDL values, while the transportation from the arterial wall to the liver is dependent on HDL values. It has also been postulated that HDL can have other protective mechanisms, such as reducing the expression of vascular adhesion molecules or an increase in endogenous fibrinolytic capacity.

Table 2. The pro-atherogenic lipid profile in RA

Low HDL and ApoA1
High ApoB/ApoA1
Hypertriglyceridemia

Table 3. Degree of evidence for the presence of the different cardiovascular risk factors and inflammatory elements in RA. ND: no data; 0: no evidence; +: moderate evidence; ++: consistent evidence

CARDIOVASCULAR RISK FACTORS/ INFLAMMATORY ELEMENTS	EVIDENCE GRADE FOR RA
Hyperinsulinemia	+
Insulin resistance	++
Trygliceridemia	+/0
Low HDL	++
Small LDL	+
Lipoprotein (a)	++
ICAM-1	++
vW Factor	+
Microalbuminuria	+
Oxidative stress	+
Fibrinogen	++
High pressure	+
Homocysteine	++
Smoking	0

Several studies have evaluated the lipid profile in RA. For example Park et al[94] observed that, in these patients, the levels of apolipoprotein (apoA) and HDL cholesterol were significantly less than in the control group. In addition, the levels of lipopoprotein(a), apoB/apoA, total cholesterol/HDL cholesterol and LDL cholesterol/HDL cholesterol ratios were significantly higher in patients with untreated RA. This reduction in HDL has also been observed in active RA and in untreated RA and in both sexes.[95] This lipid profile has also been related to inflammatory parameters, in that an inverse correlation was found between CRP and ESR with apoA and HDL cholesterol.[96]

Despite the majority of studies pointing to a pro-atherogenic profile in RA, there are studies that question this. For example, in a recent Spanish study,[96] which involved 50 patients with RA lasting more than one month and less than one year, with no previous treatment with steroids or disease modifying drugs, no statistically significant differences were found in relation to the control group. In section 2.5, the pharmacological effect of the treatment of RA on the lipid profile is discussed.

2.3.5. Insulin Resistance

Insulin resistance (IR) is defined as a defect in the action of insulin that causes an increase in basal insulin, so as to maintain glycemia within the normal range. The principal trigger is an excess of free fatty acids (FFA) derived from triglyceride reserves in the adipose tissue or from the lipolysis of lipoproteins rich in triglycerides in the tissues. On developing IR, the release of FFA in the adipose tissue increases, which, in turn, inhibits the antilipolytic effects of the insulin. Both the increase in the release of FFA and the synthesis of triglycerides are the key alterations that define this metabolic syndrome[97]

In the presence of insulin resistance, the FFA produce pro-atherogenic changes in various tissues (see Figure 10). The hyperflow of FFA to the liver produces an increase in the synthesis of triglycerides and of the triglyceride-rich VLDL (the insulin inhibiting their secretion to the circulation in physiological conditions) and apoB. This results in a decrease in the activity of the lipoprotein lipase in the adipose tissue and in the muscle, which leads to the triglycerides not being cleared from the VLDL. This stimulates the accumulation of intermediate density proteins (IDL) and LDL.

IR has also been studied in RA, the hyperinsulinemia correlating with the degree of inflammation. It has been observed that in this disease IR is produced at a muscular level more than at a hepatic level.[98] The mechanisms that have been postulated are based on the fact that the cytokines can directly impede the action of insulin at a muscle level,[99] principally by means of the TNFα. In addition, these cytokines stimulate the adipose tissue, increasing the amount of FFA and stimulating the FFA cycle between the adipose tissue and the liver.[100]

2.4. New Vascular Risk Factors

2.4.1. Homocysteine

An increasing number of epidemiological and clinical studies demonstrate that, regardless of whether a person suffers from vascular disease, a moderate increase in the plasmatic homocysteine concentration constitutes a risk factor at a coronary, cerebral and peripheral level, as well as being a risk factor for an increase in venous thrombosis.[101,102] Homocysteine contributes to the acceleration of the arteriosclerotic process. In fact, it is considered as a vascular risk factor independent of the classic risk factors. The highest correlation between hyperhomocysteinemia and arteriosclerosis occurs in peripheral vascular disease[103] and cerebrovascular disease[104] and to a lesser degree with coronary heart disease.[105]

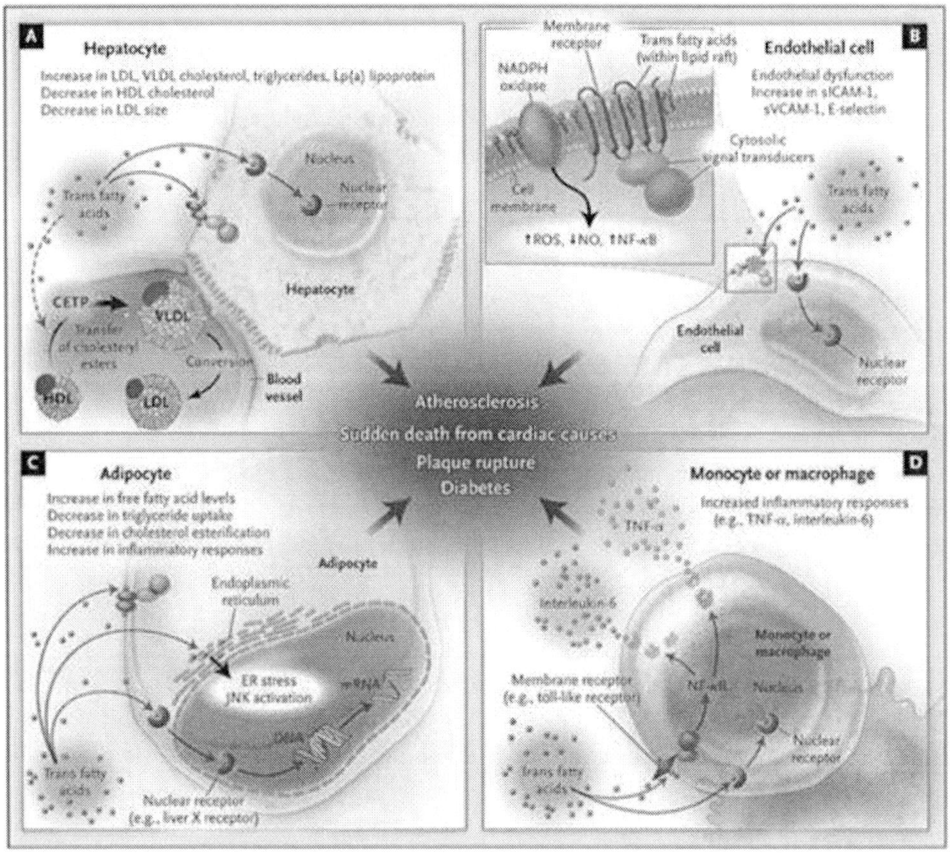

Figure 10. Resistance to insulin and the atherogenic lipoprotein profile

Homocysteine is an amino acid resulting from the action of homocysteine methyltransferase on the methionine in the diet. The homocysteine is subsequently metabolised via two pathways: trans-sulphuration, which requires the participation of vitamin B6, and transmethylation, carried out by methylenetetrahydrofolate reductase (MTHFR) which requires folate, cobalamin, and betaine homocysteine methyltransferase. Two thirds of cases of non-congenital hyperhomocysteinemia are due to a deficit of vitamins B6, B12 and folic acid.

Their pro-arteriosclerotic action occurs through various mechanisms. Homocysteine inhibits vasodilation measured by the NO and other endothelial vasodilating substances, having a direct toxic effect on endothelium and facilitating lipid peroxidation[101] . In addition, it stimulates the proliferation of smooth muscle cells and fibroblasts in blood vessels. Perhaps their most important action is their pro-thrombotic action. By interfering with the physiological anti-coagulants such as C protein and antithrombin III, it activates coagulation factors and stimulates the secretion of thromboxane A by the platelets.

In RA, high levels of homocysteine have also been found,[106] principally in relation to methotrexate, which is discussed below, as it reduces folate levels in plasma, decreasing the activity of the MTHFR.[107] It has been demonstrated that folic acid supplements in patients undergoing long-term treatment with methotrexate reduce toxicity from methotrexate and hyperhomocysteinemia. [108,109] .

The relationship between the high levels of homocysteine and inflammation in RA has also been studied. Reduced levels of vitamin B have been observed in plasma and in abnormal methionine loading test results related to high levels of inflammation markers, such as ESR, CRP, the degree of disability, matutinal rigidity and the degree of pain.[109] Finally, this relationship has also been shown in the observation of a reduction in homocysteine levels after treatment with steroid pulses. [110]

2.4.2. Lipoprotein(a)

This is a particle formed from the bonding of LDL with a glycoprotein; apoA. Although the metabolic pathways of lipoprotein(a) (Lp(a)) are not well known, it is known that the component that determines their plasmatic concentration is apoA.[111] Its function is not known, as there are people who have no Lp(a) and yet do not suffer any disease as a result.

Lp(a) levels can vary considerably, lying between 0.1 and 200 mg/dl, but they are kept constant throughout life. Even so, some studies have demonstrated a slight increase in their plasmatic concentration after myocardial infarction (MI) or a surgical operation.[112] Furthermore, an association has been observed between high plasma levels of Lp(a) and coronary heart disease.[113-115] After these findings, investigations began into the relationship of Lp(a) with the arteriosclerotic process. As a result it is beginning to be considered as an acute phase reactant.[116]

The fundamental pro-atherogenic mechanism is based on the fact the apo(a) amino acid sequence has an 80% similarity to the plasminogenic mechanism through which the apo(a) would act as a competitive inhibitor, thereby promoting the pro-thrombotic state. In addition, it stimulates the proliferation and mobility of vascular smooth muscle cells and is captured by the macrophages, giving rise to foam cells.

As discussed above, elevated Lp(a) was observed in RA patients receiving no treatment and in patients receiving active treatment. It contributes to the pro-atherogenic lipid profile and is positively correlated with high levels of CRP.[117]

2.4.3. Fibrinogen

Fibrinogen is a soluble glycoprotein synthesized at a hepatic level, the fundamental functions of which are to maintain blood viscosity, mediate platelet aggregation and intervene in the continuous haemostatic repair of the vascular endothelium and in occasional traumatic breakages.

Even so, in recent years fibrinogen has begun to be considered as a vascular risk marker,[118-125] as it has a predictive value both for ischemic heart disease and cerebrovascular disease.[122] In males, prior levels of fibrinogen constitute predictive factors for coronary heart disease, cerebrovascular accident and peripheral arterial disease. In women, fibrinogen levels correlate with coronary heart disease, peripheral arterial disease and cardiac insufficiency. It has been concluded that fibrinogen levels are related, in both sexes, to mortality of coronary origin. Various meta-analyses have been published on the relationship between fibrinogen and ischemic heart disease. However, the largest number of studies were carried out in 1998.[126] These resulted in a risk coefficient of 1.8 for ischemic heart disease in individuals with high fibrinogen.

Finally, the relationship between coronary heart disease and various components of haemostasis, as well as fibrinogen, has also been studied,[127] particularly the von Willebrand factor and the plasminogen tissue activator. However, the most important predictive factor is fibrinogen. These parameters have also been studied in patients with RA, and as already discussed in section 1.2.2.3, a pro-coagulant state has been demonstrated in this disease, principally as a consequence of fibrinogen.

2.4.4. Microalbuminuria

Microalbuminuria is defined by a urinary excretion of albumin of between 30 mmg and 300mmg in 24 hours. The Framingham study demonstrated that patients with proteinuria had a major risk of suffering from cardiovascular disease. On the basis of this, research carried out has established that microalbuminuria is a predictive factor for cardiovascular risk in AHT and diabetes.[128,129] Hypertensive patients with microalbuminuria have an increased prevalence of left ventricular hypertrophy, coronary heart disease, acute cerebrovascular accident, retinopathy and dyslipidemia, in comparison with hypertensive patients without microalbuminuria[130] .

In addition, it has been demonstrated that microalbuminuria is a cardiovascular risk factor independently of whether the patient presents diabetes or AHT. Studies have been carried out in healthy populations in which an increase in cardiovascular mortality has been observed in those with a higher urinary excretion of albumin.[131] For example, the HOPE study demonstrated an increase in the relative risk of developing a serious cardiovascular event.[132] Microalbuminuria even involved an increase in vascular risk, with a statistically significant association with hyperhomocysteinemia. [133] In RA microalbumiuria is considered to be a reflection of endothelial dysfunction, correlating with an increase in CRP in 1 out of every 4 patients.[134]

2.4.5. Oxidative Stress

As well as being pro-atherogenic, the lipid profile is also characterised by it being pro-oxidative. In RA the cytokines can directly induce oxidative modifications in the LDL, probably stimulating the secretion of super-oxides by the macrophages and endothelial cells. It has been demonstrated that lipid peroxidation and global oxidative activity is significantly increased in RA, correlating positively with acute phase reactants such as ceruloplasmin[135] but correlating inversely with anti-oxidant agents such as vitamin A and E.

2.4.6. Type B Natriuretic Peptide

Natriuretic peptides belong to a group of peptidic hormones released by myocardial cells. Three types are known: type A natriuretic peptide (ANP), the first to be identified, which is released in response to auricular dilation; type B cerebral natriuretic peptide (BNP), originating in the ventricular myocardium, which responds to increases in pressure and volume at the end of the diastole, and the type C natriuretic peptide (CNP), of endothelial origin and with functions that are still not well understood. The human BNP gene is located on chromosome 1 and codifies the prohormone of 108 pro-BNP amino acids which release the active form into the circulation i.e. the BNP of 32 amino acids, as well as the aminoterminal portion of 76 amino acids called NT-proBNP. The advantages of this over BNP are its higher blood levels in cardiac insufficiency (CI) and its major stability in circulating blood.

Determining the BNP level is useful in a variety of circumstances.[136] Its usefulness has been proved as a screening test in emergency services as a diagnostic support of CI in patients with dyspnoea of an unclear aetiology. In a study of BNP which involved 1,586 patients with acute dyspnoea, measuring BNP made it possible to differentiate between cardiac causes and non-cardiac causes, doing so with a high level of specificity and a high negative predictive value, taking a cut off point of 100 pg/ml. In fact, the European guides for the diagnosis and treatment of CI incorporate BNP as a routine test in clinical practice.

Furthermore, its usefulness has been demonstrated as a method for diagnosing asymptomatic left ventricular systolic dysfunction, although there is no consensus regarding its use in population studies. In a high-risk population (from 75 to 80 years of age), testing for BNP made the early detection of CI possible, and its measurement would be as useful, diagnostically, as a mammogram or cervical cytology. Furthermore, it can be used in the detection of subclinical vascular disease in high-risk patients. In asymptomatic hypertensive patients, BNP values have been related to left ventricular hypertrophy and both systolic and diastolic dysfunction. By contrast, regarding its determination in the Framingham population, only a third of the patients presented high levels of BNP, so its application to low vascular risk populations is questionable.

Even so, the combination of elevated levels of BNP and the presence of a long QT interval or any electrocardiographic alteration is considered to be a predictive factor, independently of undiagnosed left ventricular systolic dysfunction. This has been demonstrated with ANP, BNP and proBNP. It has also been analysed in RA. In a study of 26 patients with RA[137] with no known cardiac disease, BNP levels were significantly higher in RA patients compared to the control group and correlated with the systolic and dyastolic volume and ventricular mass in the echocardiogram. A BNP value of 5 pmol/l had a sensitivity and specificity for the detection of systolic dysfunction of 70% and 64% respectively and 60% and 69% for diastolic dysfunction.

In the future the measurement of BNP will probably cease to be used only on patients with CI. Its usefulness has been demonstrated as a short- and long-term predictor of mortality, as well as a predictor of the development of CI in patients with acute coronary syndrome without ST elevation. Furthermore, its role as a marker for cardiac transplant rejection is being studied. Finally, it is important to highlight the use of recombinant human BNP (Natrecor®) in CI, due to its diuretic, natriuretic and hypotensive effects.

2.5. The Effects of Antirheumatic Drugs on Vascular Disease

2.5.1. Non-Steroid Anti-Inflammatories

Non-steroid anti-inflammatories (NSAIDs) are widely used as analgesics for patients with RA. In addition to their analgesic effect they have a platelet anti-aggregant effect. They therefore have an important role in reducing the risk of ischemic heart disease in patients with RA. Even so, a recent study[138] observed that the risk of having a first coronary event in the two weeks after ceasing to take this medication is significant in RA and in lupus, as these patients take this form of medication discontinuously.

In addition, it is worth highlighting the importance of the new cyclo-oxygenase-2 (COX 2) inhibitors in relation to coronary risk. They selectively inhibit the production of prostaglandin E2 and prostacyclin, while they do not act on the production of thromboxane A2, an important vasoconstrictor and pro-coagulant. Their use therefore carries a potential high risk of coronary events in patients with RA. This supposition was confirmed in the

Vioxx Gastrointestinal Outcomes Research (VIGOR) study, which compared the gastrointestinal tolerance of naproxen and rofecoxib.[139] A fourfold increase in myocardial infarction was observed in the rofecoxib group.

2.5.2. Steroids

Steroids are characterised by their tendency to increase arteriosclerosis, encouraging a pro-atherogenic lipid profile, hyperglycemia and an increase in arterial pressure. Even so, they have an important anti-inflammatory effect through which, in RA, they paradoxically improve pro-arteriosclerotic inflammatory parameters. This is what is referred to as the *dual effect of steroids*. In a recent study,[140] no association was found between long-term treatment with steroids and cardiovascular events in patients with RA followed up over an average of 15 years.

In recent years, some studies have been carried out relating the use of steroids in these patients to factors that encourage accelerated arteriosclerosis. The relationship between steroids and dyslipidemia has been studied[141] in patients with stable RA, recently active RA and RA in remission after the active phase at 56 weeks of treatment with steroids and/or sulphasalazine (the COBRA study). It was observed that HDL levels were significantly higher in patients with RA in remission than in patients with active RA. There was an important reduction in the atherogenic index (total cholesterol/HDL). In addition, it has been possible to demonstrate that steroids in RA improve peripheral sensitivity to insulin due to their anti-inflammatory action.[142,143]

Furthermore, there are studies that confirm a predominance of the pro-atherogenic effects of steroids over their anti-inflammatory effects. This has been observed in studies using methods for the diagnosis of arteriosclerosis on patients at the subclinical phase, described in more detail below, principally the measurement of the intima-media thickness by carotid ultrasound. It is particularly noticeable that exposure to treatment with steroids in the long term and with high daily doses (>16 mg/day) is associated with a greater incidence of plaques observed by carotid ultrasound, and greater peripheral arterial stiffness (defined by an ankle-brachial index of >1.3).[144] However, in comparison with those patients who were not treated with corticoids, there were no differences between the two groups in either intima-media thickness or ankle-brachial index values <0.9.

2.5.3. Disease-Modifying Drugs

2.5.3.1. Methotrexate

The use of disease-modifying drugs (DMARDS), particularly methotrexate (MTX), has changed the trend that used to be observed in studies at the end of the 1980s of an increase in mortality in RA due to CD. This has been seen to have reduced in recent studies,[13] probably as a result of the introduction of new drugs in the treatment of the disease, as discussed in the introduction.

Recently studies have also been carried out which verify the importance of the use of MTX in the decrease in mortality.[145] The use of MTX is associated with a significant reduction in the risk of cardiovascular events in comparison to patients not treated with MTX. However, like steroids, MTX has a dual action, as it also has a pro-atherogenic action, increasing the levels of homocysteine,[108,109] as discussed above.

2.5.3. Other Disease-Modifying Drugs

Other drugs belonging to the disease-modifying group are anti-malarials, including particularly hydroxychloroquine, as well as sulphadiazine and cyclosporine and gold salts. Out of these, the most studied is hydroxychloroquine which stands out due to its protective role in relation to atherogenesis. This is primarily due to the change in the lipid profile, as they reduce the levels of total cholesterol and LDL.[146] The mechanism probably operates through their anti-inflammatory action, as lower levels of IL-6 have been observed in patients being treated with anti-malarials[147] .

Finally sulphadiazine, like steroids, improves insulin resistance,[142] as they both produce a significant improvement in peripheral sensitivity to insulin. In addition, sulphadiazine has been associated with hyperhomocysteinemia.[109]

2.5.4. Anti-TNF α

TNFα is the most important pro-inflammatory cytokine in the pathogenesis of RA as already discussed above. Its involvement in endothelial dysfunction, pro-atherogenic lipid profiles, lipid oxidation and the activation of other cytokines has been demonstrated. These perpetuate the inflammatory action at an arterial and endothelial level.

Currently, three anti-TNFα drugs are used in the treatment of RA: etanercept, adalimumab and infliximab. The p75 and p55 soluble receptors regulate the pro-inflammatory action of TNF, bonding with it and impeding its interaction with membrane receptors in the effector cells. *Etanercept* is composed of TNFα and TNFβ or soluble lymphotoxin α and inhibits their binding with the effector cells, impeding the pro-inflammatory process, as it is a recombinant human protein formed by the p75 receptor in its soluble form and the constant fraction (CF) of human immunoglobulin (IgG1).

By contrast, the mechanism of the other two drugs is different, as they combine both with soluble TNF α, and with the membrane and receptor. They are different in their structure. Adalimumab, like etanercept is a recombinant human IgG1 protein that combines with both the p75 and p55 receptors. By contrast, infliximab is an immunoglobulin that is 75% human in origin (the constant fraction CF) and 25% murinal (the variable fraction). In all three drugs, the results obtained are better if they are combined with disease-modifying drugs.

2.5.4.1. Antitnfα And Its Involvement In Advanced Cardiac Insufficiency

In principle, these drugs, due to their action mechanism, should substantially block the different aspects of the immune response where TNFα is the protagonist. Even so, it is difficult to evaluate their benefits at the level of the vascular inflammatory process, as a relationship between these drugs and the worsening of cardiac insufficiency has been demonstrated in functional class III and IV.

In this respect, parallel studies have been carried out with etanercept, such as the RENAISSANCE study in the United States, the RECOVER study in Europe and Australia and the RENEWAL study[148] at a global level, with patients in classes I-IV of the NYHA. In these studies there was no improvement observed in mortality rates from any cause or in relation to hospitalisations for cardiac insufficiency from taking etanercept. This relationship between anti-TNFα and cardiac insufficiency was also observed with infliximab in the ATTACH study[149,150] where patients in NYHA functional class II and IV with ejection fractions of <35% were included. It was observed that there was a dose-dependent increase in the relationship to mortality and hospitalisation due to cardiac insufficiency for those taking infliximab, in comparison with the placebo group, at week 14 and week 28 of its administration. In addition, the FDA recently received details of 47 cases of worsening or recent diagnosis of cardiac insufficiency.[148]

Finally, in a recent longitudinal study[148] of patients with RA and without cardiac insufficiency, it was observed that the incidence and prevalence of cardiac insufficiency was the same for those treated with anti-TNFα and those who were not treated with anti-TNFα. Therefore, the use of anti-TNFα should not be recommended for patients in functional class III and IV.

2.5.4.2. The Beneficial Effect Of Anti-Tnfα In Endothelial Dysfunction

Due to the important effect of TNFα on endothelial dysfunction, several studies have demonstrated a functional improvement in the endothelium after treatment with anti-TNFα for 12 weeks.[152] This includes recent studies that argue that there is a reduction in the risk of suffering a first cardiovascular event in RA patients treated with these drugs.[153]

Despite the fact that these studies support a decrease in endothelial dysfunction, what seems to be clear is that this beneficial effect is not a long-lasting. For example, a study carried out in Spain[154] showed a beneficial effect in endothelial dysfunction, evaluated by ultrasound of the brachial artery, in patients treated periodically with infliximab for 1 year. This beneficial effect was at its maximum when patients started taking the drug, but after 4 weeks of treatment the endothelial function parameters returned to their basal value.

2.5.4.3. Changes In The Pro-Atherogenic Lipid Profile Brought About By Anti-Tnfα

Studies have been published recently[155,156] describing the changes that anti-TNFα can induce in the pro-atherogenic lipid profile that characterises RA. In one of these studies,[156] the lipid profile was shown to correlate with inflammation markers after treatment with adalimumab. After two weeks of treatment, an increase in HDL cholesterol levels was observed, while the levels of LDL cholesterol had not been modified. A decrease in levels of PCR and IL-6 was also observed.

This influence of the anti-TNFα on the lipid profile has also been observed with infliximab. A study was carried out[155] with 25 patients with RA treated for a year with infliximab. A significant decrease was observed in levels of LDL cholesterol, as was an insignificant general improvement in the lipid profile (a reduction in triglycerides, total cholesterol and an increase in HDL cholesterol).

2.5.4.3 Reduced Insulin Resistance After Treatment With Anti-Tnfα

There are currently few studies that relate the use of these drugs to an improvement in insulin resistance (IR). There are observations, not yet published,[49] indicating that IR and sensitivity to insulin significantly improve in the majority of patients treated with anti-TNFα. This confirms the importance of these drugs in reducing the development of arteriosclerosis in RA.

In a Spanish study,[49] 27 patients with RA were treated with infliximab and with one or more disease modifying drugs (one of the two disease modifying drugs being methotrexate) due to the RA failing to respond to previous treatment. A significant reduction in the insulin/glucose index was observed.

2.6. The Anti-Inflammatory Effect of Statins in RA

Statins are not only useful in the treatment of dyslipidemia. It has been demonstrated that they also have an immunomodulatory and anti-inflammatory role. The mechanisms of these actions are based on their ability to modulate the maturation of T lymphocytes. They inhibit the formation of collagen in joints in animals at concentrations that do not alter the lipid profile. They suppress Th1 cells and reduce the proliferation of antiCD3/antiCD28, as well as the secretion of IFNγ by peripheral blood mononuclear cells and synovial fluid.[157] Finally, they suppress the production of pro-inflammatory cytokines in vitro after contact between macrophages and T cells. Due to these anti-inflammatory and immunomodulatory characteristics, statins improve coronary vasodilation, independently of endothelium, in patients with arteriosclerosis. [158-161]

Following on from this evidence, studies concerning the use of statins in patients with RA were carried out. The most important of these was the Trial of atorvastatin in rheumatoid arthritis (TARA),[162] carried out with 116 patients with rheumatoid arthritis who were randomised to receive 40 mg of atorvastatin or a placebo as an adjunct to existing disease-modifying anti-rheumatic drug therapy. After 6 months, the Disease Activity Score 28 (DAS 28) was recorded and levels of acute phase reactants decreased in the group treated with atorvastatin. In other studies,[163] 20mg doses of atorvastatin given over 12 weeks resulted in an improvement in arterial rigidity, particularly in patients with active RA. Other statins, such as simvastatin, reduced oxidative stress and improved endothelial function, evaluated by the flow through the brachial artery,[164,165] in patients with long term RA and normocholesterolemics.

3. Subclinical Arteriosclerosis. The Importance of Its Diagnosis in Rheumatoid Arthritis

The most frequent cause of death in western societies is cardiovascular disease, and it is for this reason that the objective of preventative measures is to bring about a reduction in the vascular risk factors that cause these diseases, through both lifestyle changes and pharmacological measures. But for these measures to be effective it is necessary to stratify the population in terms of vascular risk, in order to apply different levels of treatment to each group. For this reason, therapeutic decisions are made depending on overall risk,[165-169] which is estimated using the Framingham risk equations.[170]

In Framingham's study risk factors such as sex, age and smoking habits, together with measures such as systolic arterial pressure, total and LDL cholesterol, were combined to calculate a score that was equated to a determined risk of suffering from a coronary episode within the following 10 years. Three categories were established: a) ***High cardiovascular risk***: individuals with a >20% risk of coronary heart disease within 10 years. This group would include patients in secondary prevention programmes after an ischemic episode in any arterial area and in other similar risk situations. These situations would include those with diabetes mellitus and patients of a particular age in primary prevention programmes but with multiple risk factors. In these patients, intervention on modifiable risk factors needs to be very intense, with LDL readings reduced to <100mg/dl.[167-169] No further action is necessary to assess the risk of coronary heart disease. b) At the other extreme are ***intervals with no risk factors***, or with only one, a low Framingham score and a risk of suffering from a coronary episode in the following 10 years of <10%. These individuals have a low risk of suffering from a cardiovascular episode in both the short and long term[171] and do not need further assessment.

Lying between these two extremes is Framingham's third category of global risk, **intermediate risk**, which includes the largest segment of the population in the West. It includes individuals in primary prevention programmes with more than one risk factor for coronary heart disease, or those with only one but who are of an age for the risk to be significant. This category corresponds to an overall risk of suffering from coronary heart disease within 10 years of between 10% and 20%, and includes **subclinical arteriosclerosis**.

Individuals included in this group not only have an intermediate global risk but also present significant *individual differences*, which leads to very real uncertainty over the true individual risk. It is therefore this group of individuals who could benefit from being further stratified through the use of exploratory tests that are feasible, practical and effective, do not require blood and can evaluate the exposure of the arteries to the total vascular risk factor load.

It is important to emphasise that there is sufficient scientific evidence[180] of the predictive value of the findings of the various techniques used to diagnose subclinical arteriosclerosis or silent ischemia to be able to recommend their use on patients at intermediate global risk. Should the tests reveal an underlying pathology, there is also sufficient evidence to consider the individual to be at high risk, equivalent to those in a secondary prevention programme. On the other hand, should the tests reveal an absence of subclinical arteriosclerosis, this can be useful in reducing the intensity of treatment and reclassifying the individual as low risk.

These diagnostic techniques for subclinical arteriosclerosis have also been applied to autoimmune disease, primarily lupus and RA, both in the carotid, coronary, and peripheral arterial areas. Techniques used include the use of carotid ultrasound, the measurement of coronary calcium, CT scan and the measurement of the ankle-brachial index. These are described below.

4. Diagnostic Methods for Subclinical Arteriosclerosis

4.1. Ankle Brachial Index (ABI)

The evaluation of the presence of peripheral obstructive arterial disease (PAD) is very important, as various studies have demonstrated that subjects with PAD of the lower limbs, though asymptomatic, have a high prevalence of coronary heart disease and, to a lesser extent, cerebrovascular disease.[173-176] Furthermore, in patients with ischemic heart disease, a pathological ABI is related to a greater degree and seriousness of coronary arteriosclerosis.[177]

In recent years the significance of an ABI of < 0.9 has been studied. It has been demonstrated that carotid ultrasound shows these subjects to have a larger number of atheromatous lesions, a greater intima-media thickness (IMT)[177,180] and a higher prevalence of carotid stenosis. The majority of the studies have also found that a pathological ABI is associated with traditional vascular risk factors, finding a greater prevalence above all in relation to age and also to diabetes, smoking and high arterial pressure.[175-178,181-183] Finally, a pathological ABI is associated with higher total mortality, as a consequence of mortality of cardiac origin,[184-187] ICTUS,[188-190] and a greater incidence of coronary complications.[181,184] However, its prediction of cerebrovascular complications is less reliable.[184]

It is important to stress that ABI has been used to predict risk in both individuals with no previously diagnosed vascular disease and those with coronary heart disease that has already been diagnosed. It has been used with both sexes. Consequently, the use of this technique in patients with an intermediate Framingham risk score is useful in stratifying the risk so as to intensify or reduce the therapeutic approach. In relation to this, in a recent study[191] of 1,000 subjects between the ages of 69 and 79, without diabetes and with no previous clinical signs of cardiovascular disease, 6.4% presented subclinical arteriosclerosis in arteries in their lower limbs. This Figure reached 12% in individuals with high cardiovascular risk.

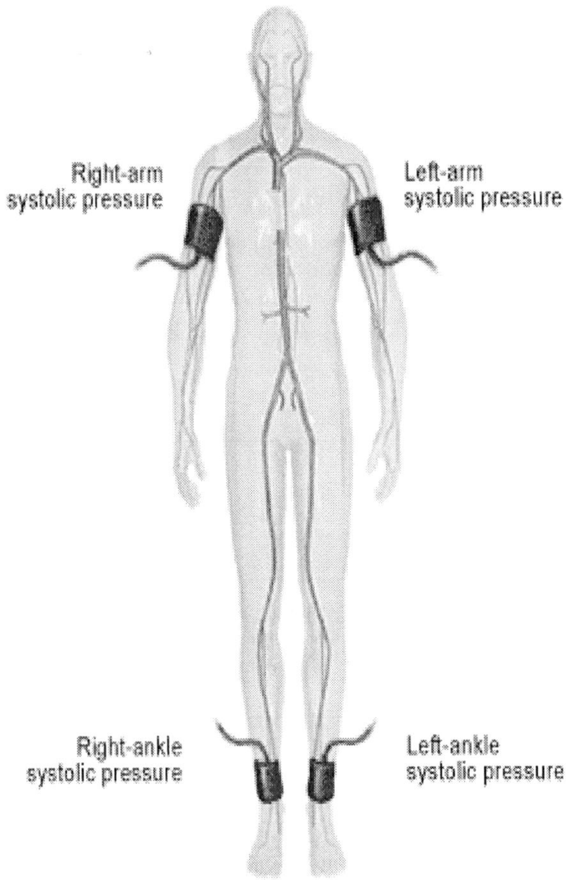

Figure 11. Methodology for calculating the ABI

Table 4. The Relationship Between Abivalues And Clinical Symptoms

	ABI	Clinical Symptoms
Normal	<1.20-1.20	Normal
Grade I	0.90-1.10	No symptoms
Grade IIa	0.90-0.60	Limb pain 200-600m
Grade IIb	0.60-0.40	Limb pain 50-200m
Grade III	0.40-0.20	Pain while resting
Grade IV	<0.20	Atrophy skin injury

4.2. Carotid Ultrasound

Carotid ultrasound (in real time or B-mode and subsequently with colour Doppler) is an economical, precise, repeatable method for the bloodless evaluation of the lumen and walls of the major arteries, allowing the *in vivo* evaluation of the early stages of cerebrovascular arteriosclerosis. The majority of studies have been carried out in the area of the carotid because of its greater accessibility. The two parameters that provide the best prediction of risk are intima-medial thickness (IMT) (see Figure 12) and the presence of atheromatous plaques (see Figure 18).

IMT is defined as the actual distance between the vascular-intima light interface and the media-adventitia interface which is better defined in the posterior arterial wall (see methods section). Studies have been carried out on healthy individuals,[192] so as to define the IMT cut off point and to establish what would constitute a normal value and what would be a pathological value. These resulted in the consideration of a measurement above the 75th percentile for age and sex to be considered as pathological, with age being the principal determining factor for IMT progression. This progression also correlates with LDL, body mass index and age.

The IMT is important as it reflects the vascular risk factor load. Various prospective studies of asymptomatic individuals of over 45 years of age have demonstrated that the IMT is a risk factor independent of the incidence of coronary heart disease [193-198] and cerebrovascular accident. [193,195,199,200]

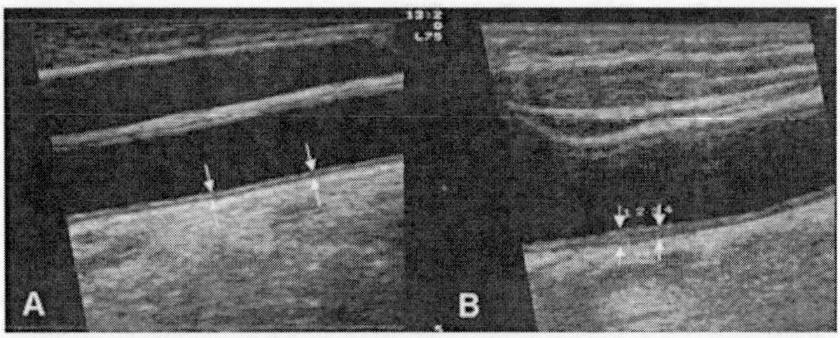

Figure 12. Intima-medial thickness (IMT). A normal IMT; B Increased IMT (corresponding to an ultrasound of a fatty streak)

In addition, various studies have evaluated the effects of treatment with statins[201,202] in the progression or regression of arteriosclerosis of the carotid arteries according to variations in IMT values. The results of these intervention studies all demonstrated that the modification of risk factors could produce significant measurable changes at an arterial level. Therefore, the usefulness of the IMT as a vascular marker in the progression and regression of the plaque, as well as its benefits in the therapeutic situation, were demonstrated.

In addition to the IMT, carotid ultrasound also allows the measurement of the number, height and size of ***atheromatous plaques*** (thickening of the IMT at a height of >1.2mm or more than 50% of the adjacent IMT) as indicators of more advanced disease (see Figure 18 and methods section). In those studies demonstrating evidence of the presence of plaques, an IMT greater than that measured when no plaques are present is always observed. It is therefore suggested that the mere detection of an increased IMT is a high-risk factor.[190,191]

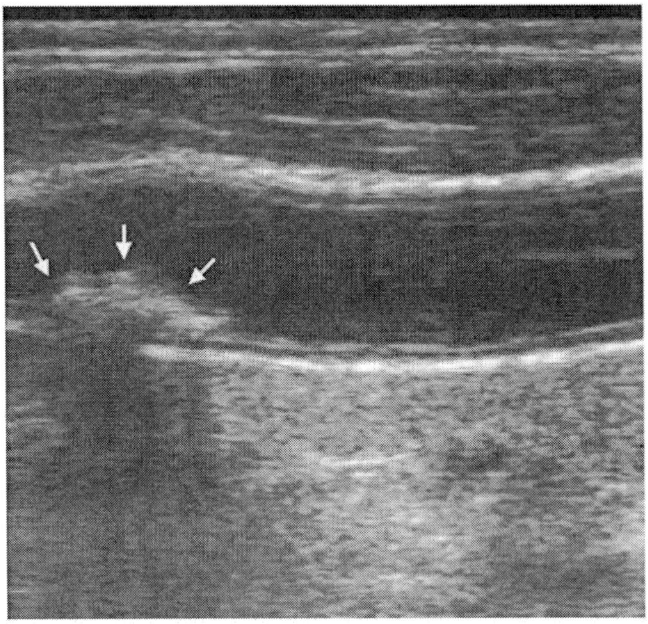

Figure 13. B-mode ultrasound. Hypoechogenic plaque on the posterior wall of the primitive carotid artery with clear calcification causing a posterior acoustic shadow

Using ultrasound, the composition of the plaques and their susceptibility to break off and form embolisms can also be determined. Hyperechogenic lesions (see Figure 13), indicating fibrosis and mineralisation (stable plaques), and hypoechogenic plaques characterised by their lipid contents, haemorrhage or necrotic tissue (unstable plaques) can also be determined. The detection of plaques that occlude >25% of the lumen of a carotid artery is considered to be a high risk.

Carotid ultrasound therefore provides a timely snapshot of the cumulative effects of all the cardiovascular risk factors affecting the arterial tree, minimising uncertainty due to individual variability. Those studies that have been carried out, both where the IMT was increased or atheromatous plaques were detected, indicated a risk of cardiovascular disease. The use of carotid ultrasound is considered to have greater predictive value than traditional risk factors in predicting vascular risk. Its use is therefore considered to be a highly valid way of stratifying individuals at risk of cardiovascular disease into low, medium or high-risk categories and thereby providing a basis on which to increase or reduce treatment.

4.3. Quantification of Coronary Calcium by Computerised Axial Tomography

The calcification of the arteries is considered, in itself, to be a risk factor for death in patients with cardiac disease.[203,204] It is associated with advanced arteriosclerosis, so patients with high calcium levels in their coronary arteries are more likely to present clinical symptoms of the disease than those with lower levels of calcification.[205]

In recent years, attempts have been made to determine whether the detection of coronary calcification by CT scan can be considered as a haemodynamically significant marker of stenosis compared with cardiac ultrasound. For these studies, conventional CT scans, electron beam CT scans and multi-cut CT scans were used. A study carried out on patients suspected of having coronary artery disease showed that 80% of the 121 patients who demonstrated significant stenosis in the cardiac ultrasound also showed calcification of the coronary arteries when examined by CT scan.[206]

These findings have also been observed in asymptomatic individuals. For example, in a large cohort of asymptomatic individuals with an average age of 53 studied with CT scans and followed-up for 3 years, a high level of coronary calcium proved to be highly predictive of coronary artery disease. The situation of these individuals is similar to that of patients in a secondary prevention programme to which it can be considered to be equivalent.[207] (See Figure 14).

As has been mentioned above, various types of CT scan have been used to study coronary calcification, although the majority have been carried out using electron beam CT scans,[208,209] which is currently thought to be the most suitable technique. To quantify coronary calcium the Agatston score algorithm (table 5), is generally used. This is a measure of surface area based on electron beam CT scans obtained with prospective gating.[208] The quantification of coronary calcium developed by Agatston is discussed in the methods section.

The volumetric quantification algorithm proposed by Callister et al is beginning to be used,[210] as it is very useful in monitoring any changes in the development of coronary artery disease because it provides good reproducibility of results in terms of quantifying surface areas.[211] As well as volumetric quantification, it also has advantages regarding surface area, considering its three-dimensional nature. As an arbitrary attenuation factor is not used, minimal variation in the attenuation area can give rise to substantial variations in the score.

The application of this technique in practice is useful in three situations. Firstly it is used in the study of atypical chest pain, as data suggests that, in patients with no previous history of coronary heart disease who attend health facilities suffering from chest pain, evaluation of calcification in the coronary arteries can be used in clinical practice as an indicator of coronary heart disease.[212] Secondly, it is used to determine the development of coronary arteriosclerosis in patients being treated with medication. Studies carried out on patients being treated with statins[210] conclude that there is a relationship between treatment with statins and LDL concentrations and the development of calcium in arteriosclerotic plaques (regression, stabilisation and progression). Finally, the most important use, as has been discussed above, is in asymptomatic individuals to stratify the risk and increase or reduce the intensity of treatment.

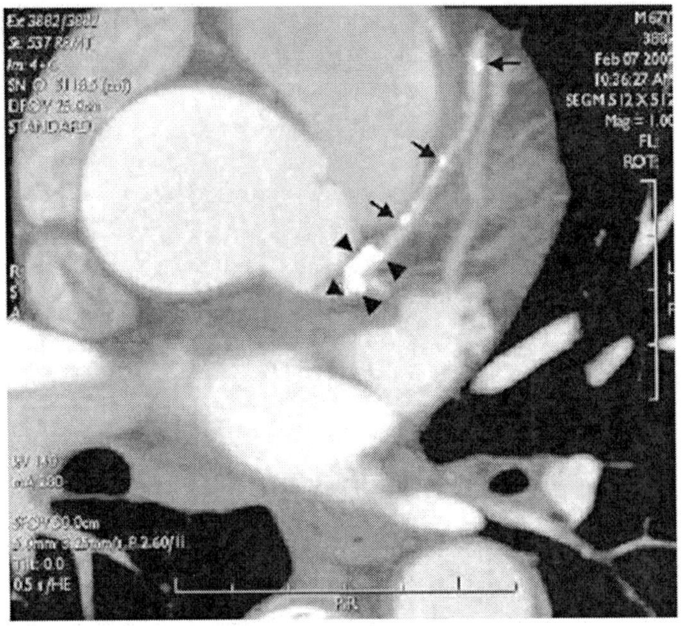

Figure 14. CT scan showing calcification of the descending anterior artery * *Reference film 61*

Table 5. Guidelines For The Interpretation Of Asymptomatic Patients According To Their Agatston Score

Value	Coronary heart disease probability	Vascular risk
0	No probability	Very low
0-10	Very low probability	Low
11-100	Low probability	Moderate
101-400	High probability	Moderate-High
>400	Significance stenosis	High

It is important to point out that this technique has significant limitations, principally that vulnerable plaques and even serious stenosis can exist in the absence of calcification.[213] Additionally, the technique is expensive and difficult to access in all centres. Even so, it is believed that: the higher the level of calcium, the greater the probability of occlusive vascular disease; the amount of total calcium correlates with the total number of arteriosclerotic plaques, and a raised level of coronary calcium correlates with a moderate to severe risk of the individual suffering from cardiovascular symptoms in the following 2 - 5 years.

5. Research into Subclinical Arteriosclerosis in AR

5.1. Peripheral Vascular Disease

A study of peripheral arteriopathy in RA has recently been carried out[214] with 243 patients with RA and 102 healthy controls. Smokers and those with a BMI of >30kg/m2 were excluded from the study. The patients with RA were found to have arterial obstruction (defined by an ABI <0.9) and a significantly greater frequency of non-compressible arteries (defined by an ABI <1.3). Patients with RA also had a greater incidence of diabetes and a significantly higher ABI.

There are studies that combine research into subclinical peripheral arterial disease with research into other arterial territories, using carotid ultrasound and electrocardiograms. For example, in a study[215] with 40 patients with RA and with no known cardiovascular risk factors, compared with healthy controls, it was found that that the proportion of people with an ABI of <1 was significantly greater in the RA group. Another study, [144] with 647 patients with RA but without a control group, evaluated the effect of corticoids both in subclinical peripheral arteriopathy and in carotid arteriopathy. Non-compressible arteries (defined as ABI>1.3) were observed more frequently in those patients who were taking steroids at doses of >16 mg every day than in those who had never taken steroids.

5.2. Carotid Disease

The use of carotid ultrasound in the study of arteriosclerotic lesions in autoimmune diseases began at the end of the 1990s, primarily in systemic lupus erythematosus (SLE).[216-222] These studies all highlighted a greater prevalence of atheromatous plaques and an increased IMT in patients with SLE than occurred in the control groups. Thus older age, the existence of previous coronary events, GGL and high systolic pressure were related to a more serious build-up of plaques. In addition, the increase in IMT has also been associated with advanced age, as well as with high systolic pressure and a high score in the SLE damage index (Lupus International Collaborating Clinics - SLICC) which evaluates the chronic organic lesions produced by the disease. Furthermore, no correlation has been found with either the use of prednisone or the presence of antiphospholipid antibodies.

A recent study[222] of 197 patients with SLE and a control group confirmed that the presence of atheromatous plaques was more prevalent in patients with SLE. Only the presence of this disease, advanced age, and the high levels of cholesterol were independent factors associated with the presence of plaques. In addition, when comparing those subjects in the SLE group who had atheromatous plaques with those who did not, findings from previous studies were confirmed i.e. a positive correlation with the duration of the disease, a higher score on the SLICC index and less treatment with immunosuppressants, which suggests that chronic inflammation plays an important role as an atherogenic mechanism.

The use of carotid ultrasound in RA began a few years after its use in SLE. Several studies were carried out at the beginning of the 21st century.[223] The majority of these studies demonstrated the duration of the disease to be the factor that was most associated with an increase in IMT and the presence of atherometous plaques. For example, in a study[224] carried out with 47 patients with RA, compared with a healthy control group, an increased IMT and the presence of a significant quantity of atheromatous plaques in patients with RA was observed. Age, greater extra-articular involvement and the disease development time were found to be the major predictors of morphological changes in the carotid. Three other studies,[225,226,215] with no significant differences related to the vascular risk factors, reached the same conclusions.

Additionally, a recent study[227] evaluated the presence of atheromatous plaques in 101 patients with SLE, 80 patients with RA (both with no known previous history of vascular disease) and 105 healthy controls. The prevalence of atheromatous plaques was greater in patients with SLE and RA than in the control group, as were radial artery tonometry measurements, despite the fact that the controls presented significantly more vascular risk factors. In patients with both diseases, this was associated with inflammatory parameters such as CRP and IL-6.

The studies discussed above excluded patients with RA who had a previous diagnosis of vascular risk factors, so that in recent years the true vascular risk that is intrinsic to RA has begun to be evaluated. For example, in a study[228] comparing 204 patients with RA with 102 in a control group, an increase in IMT and the presence of atheromatous plaques was observed in the patients suffering from RA. In this group there were also more patients with diabetes and more patients who were significantly obese compared with the control group. The increase in IMT was associated with an increase in the erythrocyte sedimentation rate (ESR) in both groups and, because of this, the possibility that vascular risk factors were more important than RA in the changes observed in the carotid began to be evaluated.

This relationship between morphological changes and the inflammatory parameters was also evaluated in patients with RA, without comparing the results with a control group. In a study of 603 patients with RA,[229] without excluding those with previously known vascular risk factors, 11-16% of the variation in IMT and the presence of atheromatous plaques was explained by demographic factors, such as age and duration of disease, 4-12% by vascular risk factors and 1-6% by factors intrinsic to the actual disease, above all in the young. It was also noted that the greater the vascular risk factors the higher the ESR. On comparing patients with and without atheromatous plaques it was discovered that those with plaques were more likely to have arterial hypertension, diabetes and hypercholesterolemia.

Following this line of research, various studies have been carried out that did not find a significant relationship between increased IMT and the presence of RA. Instead, a relationship was found between increased IMT and vascular risk factors such as age and dyslipidemia [230] (both in the carotid and femoral arteries). In another study,[231] the vascular risk factors were so significant that the IMT was greater in the control group, and although there were significant differences between the groups in relation to the presence of atheromatous plaques, the patients with RA who presented with plaques were significantly more likely to be older, smoke more and suffer from arterial hypertension and hypercholesterolemia.

There are studies that relate IMT and atheromatous plaques to the medication used to treat the disease. In a study described above,[144] the use of glucocorticoids and known vascular risk factors in 647 patients with RA were evaluated in relation to the presence of peripheral arterial disease and subclinical carotid disease. In examining the incidence of carotid disease, out of those patients who had not received steroids (34% of the sample), 47% had atheromatous plaques, while out of those who had received corticoids at a dose of >16 mg/ per day, 62% presented plaques. Similarly, another study[231] demonstrated that the presence of plaques in patients with RA is significantly related with the use of anti TNFα. This relationship can be explained if we see the greater use of immunosuppressants as a marker of disease severity and activity. The next step is to analyse the development of IMT and atheromatous plaques after using alternative treatments, such a DMARDS and NSAIDS, after a specified period of time.

5.3. Coronary Heart Disease

As discussed above, CT scans are expensive and difficult for most centres to access, unlike carotid ultrasound. Very few studies therefore use CT scans in SLE and RA.

Of the studies of SLE, two are particularly worth mentioning. The first, carried out in 1999[232] had a sample size of only 13 patients who had SLE plus two or more vascular risk factors, and a control group. The results cannot therefore be evaluated. By contrast, in a recent study[233] coronary calcium was measured in 65 patients with SLE with no history of coronary heart disease but with known vascular risk factors and with an average age of 40 and compared to a control group of 69 people. It was found that coronary calcification, measured using the Agatston score, was greater in patients with SLE with an average Agatston score of 68, compared to a score of 8 in the control group. Only in 7 patients with SLE was the score >100. Among the patients with SLE, the duration of the disease did not have a statistically significant influence on the presence or absence of coronary calcification, but age and being male did. The difference in both groups can be explained not only by the inflammatory factor intrinsic to SLE; vascular risk factors could also play an important role in the increased Agatston score. In this study, patients with SLE had a greater prevalence of hypertension, smoking and family history of cardiovascular disease than the control group.

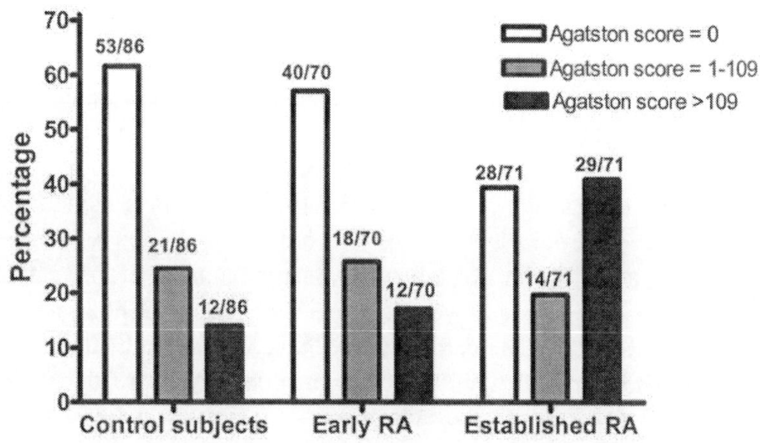

Figure 15. Distribution of the quantification of coronary calcium by CT scan in patients with recently diagnosed RA, established RA and the control group. * *Reference film 234*

In relation to RA, a recent study [234] compared the prevalence and severity of coronary arteriosclerosis evaluated by coronary calcification in patients with recently diagnosed RA (<5 years duration) (70 patients), patients with established RA (>10 duration) (71 patients) and a control group (86 patients). The patients with established RA were older and presented criteria for arterial hypertension more frequently than the other groups . The lipid profile was similar across the three groups. It was observed that the average Agatston score was significantly higher in patients with established RA in comparison with the other two groups (see Figure 20). In addition, coronary calcification was more prevalent in patients with established RA (60.6%) than in patients with recently diagnosed RA (42.9%) and the control group (38.4%), such that the odds ratio for having severe coronary calcification (defined by an Agatston score of >109) in patients with established RA was 3.42 (see Figure 15).

5.4. Electrocardiographic Alterations

It is well established that the degree of dispersion of QT represents an increase in susceptibility to ventricular tachyarrhythmia and sudden death. It is therefore important to classify them in the study of any heart disease. This parameter has also been studied in the evaluation of subclinical heart disease in RA. The mechanism through which these alterations in cardiac rhythm are produced in RA is not well understood. It is postulated that they could be related to the presence of rheumatoid nodules or inflammatory lesions in the myocardium, as well as to vasculitis and coronary arteriosclerosis.

Various studies used both the QT dispersion (QTd) (defined as the difference between the maximum and minimum QT) and the QT interval corrected for heart rate (QTc) (see the methods section). One study[235] carried out with 42 RA patients with no known heart disease compared with a healthy control group concluded that both the QTd and the QTc were significantly greater in patients with RA. Furthermore, another study carried out in 2002,[236] with 40 patients with RA and the same controls also reached the same conclusion. In relation to the previous study it added that both the QTd and the QTc were greater in those patients with RA of more than 5 years development, and related these electrocardiographic alterations to the length of time the disease had been developing. An echocardiographic analysis was also carried out, and concluded that the diastolic dysfunction parameters were altered more significantly in patients with RA, principally in those patients who had been developing the disease for longer.

However, in addition to evaluating the degree of QT dispersion another type of arrhythmia has been evaluated, with contradictory results. In this study, referred to previously,[235] Holter electrocardiograms were recorded over 24 hours. It was observed that the majority of the patients with RA showed a large number of premature ventricular complexes. By contrast, another study was also carried out using 24-hour electrocardiograms with 70 patients with RA.[237] The cardiac arrhythmias found were similar to those of the control group and did not correlate with the development of RA, its treatment, the presence of rheumatoid factor, or with extra-articular indications.

Finally, as already discussed in the two sections above, a study [215] evaluated the QT interval along with peripheral and carotid arteriopathy. A significantly higher QTd was observed in patients with RA, principally in those who were taking steroids.

References

[1] Markenson, JA. Worlwide trends in the socioeconomic impact and long-term prognosis of rheumatoid arthritis. *Semin Arthritis Rheum*, 1991, 21(Supl 1), 4-12.

[2] Paredes, S; Masana, L. Mortalidad global y por enfermedad cardiovascular en pacientes con artritis reumatoide. Clínica e Investigación en *Arteriosclerosis,* 2001, 13(2), 70-79

[3] Reilly, P; Cosh, J; Maddison, P; Rasker, J; Silman, A. Mortality and survival in rheumatoid arthritis: a 25 years prospective study of 100, patients. *Ann Rheum Dis.,* 1990, 49, 363-369.

[4] Van Doornum, S; McColl, I; Wicks, P. Accelerated atherosclerosis: An extraarticular feature of rheumatoid arthritis?. *Arthritis Rheum,* 2002, 46(4), 862-73.

[5] Sattar, N; Mc Carey, DW; Capell, H. Explaining how "high grade" systemic inflammation accelerates vascular risk in rheumatoid arthritis. Circulation, 2003, 108, 2957-2963.

[6] Guedes, C; Dumont-Fischer, D; Leichter-Nakache, S; Boissier, MC. Mortality in rheumatoid arthritis. *Rev Rhum Engl Ed.,* 1999, 66, 492-8.

[7] Pincus, T; Callahan, LF. Rheumatology function tests: grip strength, walking time, button test and questionnaires document and predict longterm morbidity and mortality in rheumatoid arthritis. *J Rheumatol,* 1992, 19, 1051-7.

[8] Pincus, T; Callahan, LF. Taking mortality in rheumatoid arthritis seriously predictive markers, socioeconomic status and comorbidity. *J Rheumatol,* 1986, 13, 841-5.

[9] Mutru, O; Laakso, M; Isomaki, H; Koota, K. Ten year mortality and causes of death in patients with rheumatoid arthritis. *Br Med J,* (Clin Res Ed) 1985, 290, 1797-9.

[10] Wolfe, F; Mitchell, D; Sibley, J; Fries, J; Bloch, D; Williams, C; et al. The mortality of rheumatoid arthritis. *Arthritis Rheum*, 1994, 37, 481-494.

[11] Wallberg-Jonsson, S; Öhman, M; Dahlqvist, S. Cardiovascular morbility and mortality in patients with seropositive rheumatoid arthritis in Northern Sweden. *J Rheumatol,* 1997, 24, 445-451.

[12] Maradit-Kremers, H; Nicola, PJ; Crowson Karla, V; Ballman Sherine, EG. Cardiovascular death in rheumatoid arthritis: a population-based study. *Arthritis Rheum,* 2005, 52(3), 722-32.

[13] Krishnan, E; Phil, L; Vijaya, B; Singh, G. Declines in Mortality From Acute Myocardial Infarction in Successive Incidence and Birth Cohorts of Patients with Rheumatoid Arthritis. *Circulation*, 2004, 110(13), 1774-1779.

[14] Jiménez, S; Font, J; Ingelmo, M. Lupus eritematoso sistémico y enfermedad cardiovascular. *MedClin*, (Barc) 2002, 119(18), 699-706.

[15] Urowitz, MB; Bookman, AM; Koehler, BE; Smythe, HA; Ogryzlo, MA. The bimodal pattern of systemic lupus erythematosus. *Am J Med.*, 1976, 60, 221-5.

[16] Stähl-Hallengren, C; Jönsen, A; Niven, O; Sturfelt, G. Incidence studies of systemic lupus erythematosus in Southern Sweden: increasing age; deceasing frequency of renal manifestations and good prognosis. *J Rheumatol,* 2000, 3, 685-91.

[17] Font, J; Ramos-Casals, M; Cervera, R; García-Carrasco, M; Torras, A; Sisó, A; et al. Cardiovascular risk factors and the long term outcome of lupus nephritis. *QJ Med.*, 2001, 94, 19-26.

[18] Mangas, A; Toro, R; Cano, S; Barba, A. Patogenia de la arteriosclerosis. Mecanismos celulares y moleculares implicados en la aterogénesis. *Medicine*, 2005, 9(38), 2495-2505.

[19] Badimon, JJ; Badimon, L; Fuster, V. Fisiopatología de la enfermedad aterotrombótica coronaria. *Clin Invest Arterioscl,* 2002, 14(5), 258-71.

[20] Göran, K. Hansson. Inflammation; Atherosclerosis; and Coronary Artery Disease. *N Engl J Med.*, 2005, 352, 1685-95.

[21] Ross, R. Atherosclerosis. An Inflammatory Disease. *N Engl Med*, 1999, 340(2), 115-123.

[22] Padró, T; Mendieta, C; Badimon, L. Inflamación y arteriosclerosis. *Hipertensión*, 2005, 22(4), 173-82.

[23] Van Albada-Kuipers, G; Brujn, J; Westedt, M; Breedveld, F; Eulderink, F. Coronary arteritis complicating rheumatoid arthritis. *Ann Rheum Dis*, 1986, 45, 963-965.

[24] Karten, I. Arteritis; myocardial infarction and rheumatoid arthritis. *JAMA*, 1969, 210, 1717-1720.

[25] Bjornadal, L. Impact of parental history on patients cardiovascular mortality in rheumatoid arthritis. *Ann Rheum Dis.*, 2006, 65(6), 741-5.

[26] Ku, DN; Giddens, DP; Zarins, CK; Glagov, S. Pulsatile flow and atherosclerosis in the human carotid bifurcation: positive correlation between plaque location and low oscillating shear stress. *Arteriosclerosis,* 1985, 5, 293-302.

[27] Malek, AM; Alper, SL; Izunmo, S. Hemodynamic shear stress and its role in atherosclerosis. *JAMA,* 1999, 282, 2035-42.

[28] Camejo, G; Hurt-Camejo, E; Wiklund, O; Bondjers, G. Association of apo B lipoproteins with arterial proteoglycans: pathological significance and molecular basis. *Atherosclerosis.,* 1998, 139, 205-22.

[29] Khera, A; James, A; Peshock, R; Hao, S; Stanek, H; Murphy, S. Relationship Between C-Reactive Protein and Subclinical Atherosclerosis: The Dallas Heart Study. *Circulation*, 2006, 113(1), 38-43.

[30] Virmani, R; Kolodgie, FD; Burke, AP; Farb, A; Schwartz, SM. Lessons from sudden coronary death: a comprehensive morphological classification scheme for atherosclerotic lesions. Arterioscler Thromb *Vasc Biol.* 2000, 20, 1262-75.

[31] Duverger, N; Kruth, H; Emmanuel, F; Caillaud, JM; Viglietta, C; Castro, G; et al. Inhibition of atherosclerosis development in cholesterol-fed human apolipoprotein A-I-transgenic rabbits. *Circulation*, 1996, 94, 713-7.

[32] Bennett, MR. Apoptosis of vascular smooth muscle cells in vascular remodelling and atherosclerotic plaque rupture. *Cardiovasc Res.*, 1999, 41, 361-8.

[33] Geng, YJ; Henderson, LE; Levesque, EB; Muszynski, M; Libby, P. Fas is expressed in human atherosclerotic intima and promotes apoptosis of cytokine-primed human vascular smooth muscle cells. *Arterioscler Thromb Vasc Biol.*, 1997, 17, 2200-8.

[34] Kolodgie, FD; Narula, J; Haider, N; Virmani, R. Apoptosis in atherosclerosis. Does it contribute to plaque instability?. *Cardiol Clin*, 2001, 19, 127-39.

[35] Sattar, N; McCarey, D; Capell, H; McInnes, I. Explaining How "High-Grade" Systemic Inflammation Accelerates Vascular Risk in Rheumatoid Arthritis. *Circulation*, 2003, 108(24), 2957-2963.

[36] Edward, TH. CRP as a Mediator of Disease. *Circulation*, 2004, 109(21) SupplementII: 11-14

[37] Gómez Jerique, JA. Inflamación; hemostasia y enfermedad coronaria. La proteína C reactiva y el dímero D como marcadores del proceso de la arteriosclerosis. *Clin Invest Arterioscl,* 2002, 14(5).242-57.

[38] Hashimoto, H; Kitagawa, K; Hougaku, H; Shimizu, Y; Sakaguchi, M; Nagai, Y; Iyama, S; Yamanishi, H; Matsumoto, M; Hori, M. C-Reactive Protein Is an Independent Predictor of the Rate of Increase in Early *Carotid Atherosclerosis. Circulation,* 2001, 104(1), 63-67.

[39] Healy, H; Westhuyzen, J. Biology and relevance of C-reactive protein in cardiovascular and renal disease. *Ann Clin Lab Sci,* 2000, 30, 133-43.

[40] Virchow, R. Phlogose und thrombose im Gefa system. En: Virchow R; editor. Gesammelte Abhandlungen zur wissenschaftliche Medizin. *Berlin: Meidinger Sohn,* 1856, 458-63.

[41] Tracy, RP. Inflammation markers and coronary heart disease. *Curr Opin Lipidol,* 1999, 10, 345-441.

[42] Danesh, J; Whincup, P; Walker, M; Lennon, L; Thomson, A; Appleby, P; et al. Low grade inflammation and coronary heart disease: prospective study and updated meta-analyses. BMJ, 2000, 321, 199-204.

[43] Blake, G; Ridker, PM. Novel clinical markers of vascular wall inflammation. *Circ Res.,* 2001, 89, 763-71.

[44] Cleland, SJ; Sattar, N; Petrie, JR; Forouhi, NG; Elliot, HL; Connell, JMC. Endothelial dysfunction as a possible link between C-reactive protein levels and cardiovascular disease. *Clin Sci.,* 2000, 98, 531-5.

[45] Molenaar, ETH; Voskuyl, AE; Familian, A; Van Mierlo, GJ; Dijkmans, BAC; Hack, CE. Complement activation in patients with rheumatoid arthritis mediated in part by C-reactive protein. *Arthritis Rheum,* 2001, 44, 997-1002.

[46] Urieli-Shoval, S; Linke, RP; Matzner, Y. Expression and function of serum amyloid A; a major acute-phase protein; in normal and disease states. *Curr Opin Hematol,* 2000, 7, 64-9.

[47] Meek, RL; Urieli-Shoval, S; Benditt, EP. Expression of apolipoprotein serum amyloid A mRNA in human atherosclerotic lesions and cultured vascular cells: implications for serum amyloid A function. Proc Natl *Acad Sci.,* 1994, 91, 3186-90.

[48] Liuzzo, G; Goronzy, JJ; Yang, H; Kopecky, SL; Holmes, DR; Frye, RL; Weyand, CM. Monoclonal T-cell proliferation and plaque instability in acute coronary syndromes. *Circulation,* 2000, 101, 2883–2888.

[49] Gonzalez-Gay, MA. Rheumatoid arthritis: a disease associated with accelerated atherogenesis. Semin *Arthritis Rheum,* 2005, 35(1), 8-17.

[50] Clancy, RM; Amin, AR; Abramson, SB. The role of nitric oxide in inflammation and immunity. *Arthritis Rheum,* 1998, 41, 1141–1151.

[51] St Clair, WE; Wilkinson, T; Lang, L; Sanders, MA. Increased expression of blood mononuclear cell nitric oxide synthase type 2 in rheumatoid arthritis; *J Exp Med.*, 1996, 184, 1173–1178.

[52] Yki-Jarkiven, R. Increased inflammatory activity parallels increased basal nitric oxide production and blunted response to nitric oxide in vivo in rheumatoid arthritis; *Ann Rheum Dis.,* 2003, 62, 630–634.

[53] Van't Hof, L; Hocking; PK. Nitric oxide is a mediator of apoptosis in the rheumatoid joint. *Rheumatology*, 2000, 39, 1004–1008.

[54] Kolb, H. Nitric oxide in autoimmune disease: cytotoxic or regulatory mediator?; *Immunol Today,* 1998, 19, 556–561.

[55] Gonzalez-Gay, MA; Llorca, J; Sanchez, E. Inducible but not endothelial nitric oxide synthase polymorphism is associated with susceptibility to rheumatoid arthritis in northwest Spain; *Rheumatology*, (Oxford) 2044, 43, 1182-1185.

[56] Glosli, H; Tronstad, KJ; Wergedal, H. Human TNF-α in transgenic mice induces differential changes in redox status and glutathione-regulating enzymes; *FASEB J.*, 2002, 16, 1450–1452.

[57] Hermann, C; Assmus, B; Urbich, C; Zeiher, AM. Insulin-mediated stimulation of protein kinase Akt: a potent survival signaling cascade for endothelial cells; *Arterioscler Thromb Vasc Biol.*, 2000, 20, 402–409.

[58] Yoshizumi, MA; Perrella, JC. Tumor necrosis factor down regulates an endothelial nitric oxide synthase mRNA by shortening its half-life; *Circ Res.,* 1993, 73, 205–209.

[59] Bloom, BJ; Miller, LC; Tucker, LB; et al. Soluble adhesion molecules in juvenile rheumatoid arthritis. *J Rheumatol.,* 1999, 26 2044–2048.

[60] Veale, DJ; Maple, C; Kirk, G; et al. Soluble cell adhesion molecules–P-selectin and ICAM-1, and disease activity in patients receiving sulphasalazine for active rheumatoid arthritis. Scand *J Rheumatol.,* 1998, 27, 296–299.

[61] Ros, E; Zambón, D; Gilabert, R. Técnicas de diagnóstico de aterosclerosis preclínica y su utilización para mejorar la predicción de riesgo cardiovascular. *Clin Invest Arterioscl.,* 2002, 14(4), 187-97.

[62] Gonzalez-Juanatey, C; Testa, A; Garcia-Castelo, A; Garcia-Porrua, C. HLA-DRB1 status affects endothelial function in treated patients with rheumatoid arthritis; *Am J Med.*, 2003, 114, 647–652.

[63] Vaudo, G; Marchesi, S; Gerli, R; Allegrucci, R; Giordano, A. Endothelial dysfunction in young patients with rheumatoid arthritis and low disease activity; *Ann Rheum Dis.,* 2004, 63, 31–35.

[64] Grisar, J. Depletion of Endothelial Progenitor Cells in the Peripheral Blood of Patients With Rheumatoid Arthritis. *Circulation*, 2005, 111(2), 204-211.

[65] Morishita, Y; Sao, H; Hansen, JA; Martin, PJ. A distinct subset of human CD4+ cells with a limited alloreactive T cell receptor repertoire. *J Immunol.*, 1989, 143, 2783–2789.

[66] Markovic-Plese, S; Cortese, I; Wandinger, KP; McFarland, HF; Marti, R. CD4+CD28- costimulation-independent T cells in multiple sclerosis. *J Clin Invest.*, 2001, 108, 1185–1194.

[67] Lamprecht, P; Moosig, F; Csernok, E; Seitzer, U; Schnabel, A; Mueller, A; Gross, WL. CD28 negative T cells are enriched in granulomatous lesions the respiratory tract in Wegener's granulomatosis. *Thorax*, 2001, 56, 751-757.

[68] Martens, PB; Goronzy, JJ; Schaid, D; Weyand, CM. Expansion of unusual CD4+ T cells in severe rheumatoid arthritis. *Arthritis Rheum,* 1997, 40, 1106–1114.

[69] Namekawa, T; Wagner, UG; Goronzy, JJ; Weyand, CM. Functional subsets of CD4 T cells in rheumatoid synovitis. *Arthritis Rheum.,* 1998, 41, 2108–2116.

[70] Schmidt, D; Martens, PB; Weyand, CM; Goronzy, JJ. The repertoire of CD4+ CD28-T cells in rheumatoid arthritis. *Mol Med.*, 1996, 2, 608–618.

[71] Bryl, E; Vallejo, AN; Weyand, CM; Goronzy, JJ. Down-regulation of CD28 expression by TNF-alpha. *J Immunol*, 2001, 167, 3231–3238.

[72] Park, W; Weyand, CM; Schmidt, D; Goronzy, JJ. Co-stimulatory pathways controlling activation and peripheral tolerance of human CD4+CD28- T cells. *Eur J Immunol.*, 1997, 27, 1082–1090.

[73] Schmidt, D; Goronzy, JJ; Weyand, CM. CD4+CD7-CD28- T cells are expanded in rheumatoid arthritis and are characterized by autoreactivity. *J Clin Invest.*, 1996, 97, 2027–2037.

[74] Schirmer, M; Vallejo, AN; Weyand, CM; Goronzy, JJ. Resistance to apoptosis and elevated expression of Bcl-2 in clonally expanded CD4+CD28- T cells from rheumatoid arthritis patients. *J Immunol*, 1998, 161, 1018–1025.

[75] Warrington, KJ; Takemura, S; Goronzy, JJ; Weyand, CM. CD4+CD28- T cells in rheumatoid arthritis patients combine features of the innate and adaptive immune systems. *Arthritis Rheum,* 2001, 44, 13–20.

[76] Snyder, MR; Muegge, LO; Offord, C; O'Fallon, WM; Bajzer, Z; Weyand, CM; Goronzy, JJ. Formation of the killer Ig-like receptor on CD4+CD28 null T cells. *J Immunol,* 2002, 168, 3839–3846.

[77] Libby, P; Ridker, PM; Maseri, A. Inflammation and atherosclerosis. *Circulation.,* 2002, 105, 1135–1143.

[78] Van Doornum, S; McColl, G; Wicks, IP. Accelerated atherosclerosis: an extraarticular feature of rheumatoid arthritis? *Arthritis Rheum,* 2002, 46, 862–873.

[79] Grignani, G; Maiolo, A. Cytokines and hemostasis. *Haematologica*, 2000, 85, 967–972.

[80] Aguilera, C; Aranda, A; Sánchez, JP. Análisis del perfil lipídico en pacientes con arthritis reumatoide de inicio reciente. *Med Clin*, (Barc). 2006, 127(8), 313-5.

[81] Tam, LS; Gladman, DD; Hallett, DC; Rahman, P; Urowitz, MB. Effect of antimalarial agents on the fasting lipid profile in systemic lupus erythematosus. *J Rheumatol.,* 2000, 27, 2142.

[82] Sokka, T; Mottonen, T; Hannonen, P. Mortality in early "sawtooth" treated rheumatoid arthritis patients during the first 8-14 years. Scand *J Rheumatol.,* 1999, 28, 282-7.

[83] Hazes, JM; Dijkmans, BA; Vandenbroucke, JP; de Vries, RR; Cats, A. Lifestyle and the risk of rheumatoid arthritis: cigarette smoking and alcohol consumption. *Ann Rheum Dis.,* 1990, 49, 980-2.

[84] Hernandez Avila, M; Liang, MH; Willett, WC; Stampfer, MJ; Colditz, GA; Rosner, B; et al. Reproductive factors; smoking; and the risk for rheumatoid arthritis. *Epidemiology*, 1990, 1, 285-91.

[85] Heliovaara, M; Aho, K; Aromaa, A; Knekt, P; Reunanen, A. Smoking and risk of rheumatoid arthritis. *J Rheumatol,* 1993, 20, 1830-5.

[86] Voigt, LF; Koepsell, TD; Nelson, JL; Dugowson, CE; Daling, JR. Smoking; obesity; alcohol consumption; and the risk of rheumatoid arthritis. *Epidemiology*, 1994, 5, 525-32.

[87] Silman, AJ; Newman, J; MacGregor, AJ. Cigarette smoking increases the risk of rheumatoid arthritis: results from a nationwide study of disease-discordant twins. *Arthritis Rheum.,* 1996, 39, 732-5.

[88] Symmons, DPM; Bankhead, CR; Harrison, BJ; Brennan, P; Barrett, EM; Scott, DGI; et al. Blood transfusion; smoking; and obesity as risk factors for the development of rheumatoid arthritis: results from a primary care-based incident case-control study in Norfolk; England. *Arthritis Rheum,* 1997, 40, 1955-61.

[89] Uhlig, T; Hagen, KB; Kvien, TK. Current tobacco smoking; formal education; and the risk of rheumatoid arthritis. *J Rheumatol,* 1999, 26, 47-54.

[90] Karlson, EW; Lee, IM; Cook, NR; Manson, JE; Buring, JE; Hennekens, CH. A retrospective cohort study of cigarette smoking and risk of rheumatoid arthritis in female health professionals. *Arthritis Rheum,* 1999, 42, 910-7.

[91] Hutchinson, D; Shepstone, L; Moots, R; Lear, JT; Lynch, MP. Heavy cigarette smoking is strongly associated with rheumatoid arthritis (RA); particularly in patients without a family history of RA. *Ann Rheum Dis.,* 2001, 60, 223-7.

[92] Saag, KG; Cerhan, JR; Kolluri, S; Ohashi, K; Hunninghake, GW; Schwartz, DA. Cigarette smoking and rheumatoid arthritis severity. *Ann Rheum Dis,* 1997, 56, 463-9.

[93] Wolfe, F. The effect of smoking on clinical; laboratory and radiographic status in rheumatoid arthritis. *J Rheumatol,* 2000, 27, 630-7.

[94] Park, YB; Lee, WK; Suh, CH. Lipid profiles in untreated patients with rheumatoid arthritis. *J Rheumatol,* 1999, 26, 1701-4.

[95] Lazarevic, MB; Vitic, J; Mladenovic, V; Myones, BL; Skosey, JL; Swedler, WI. Dyslipoproteinemia in the course of active rheumatoid arthritis. Semin *Arthritis Rheum,* 1992, 22, 172-8.

[96] Yoo, WH. Dyslipoproteinemia in patients with active rheumatoid arthritis: effects of disease activity; sex; and menopausl status on lipid profiles. *J Rheumatol,* 2004, 31, 1746-53.

[97] Laclaustra, M; Bergua, C; Pascual, I. Síndrome metabólico. Concepto y fisiopatología. *Rev Esp Cardiol*, 2006, 5, 3-10.

[98] Paolisso, G; Valentini, G; Giugliano, D; et al. Evidence for peripheral impaired glucose handling in patients with connective tissue diseases. *Metabolism*, 1991, 40, 902–907.

[99] Hotamisligil, GS; Peraldi, P; Budavari, A; et al. IRS-1-mediated inhibition of insulin receptor tyrosine kinase activity in TNF-alpha- and obesity-induced insulin resistance. *Science*, 1996, 271, 665–668.

[100] Chajek-Shaul, T; Friedman, G; Stein, O; et al. Mechanism of the hypertriglyceridemia induced by tumor necrosis factor administration to rats. *Biochim Biophys Acta*, 1989, 1001, 316–324.

[101] Córdoba, A; Blanco, F; González, F. Hiperhomocisteinemia: un nuevo marcador de riesgo cardiovascular: territorios vasculares afectados; papel en la patogénesis de la arterioesclerosis y la trombosis y tratamiento. *Med Clín*, 1997, 109, 715-725.

[102] Abellán, J; Hernández, F. Los nuevos factores de riesgo vascular. *Hipertensión*, 2001, 18(4), 171-183.

[103] Selhlub, J; Jacques, PF; Bostom, AG; D'Agostino, RB; Wilson, PWF; Belanger, AJ. Association between plasma homocysteine concentrations and extracranial carotid-artery stenosis. *N Engl J Med*, 1995, 332, 286-291.

[104] Perry, IJ; Refsum, H; Morris, RW; Ebrahim, SB; Ueland, PM; Shaper, AG. Prospective study of serum total homocysteine concentration and risk of stroke in middle-aged British men. *Lancet*, 1995, 346, 1.395-1.398.

[105] Stampfer, MJ; Malinow, MR; Willett, WC; Newcomer, LM; Upson, B; Ullmann, D. A prospective study of plasma homocysteine and risk of myocardial infarction in US physicians. *J Am Med Associ*, 1992, 268, 877-881.

[106] Hernanz, A; Plaza, A; Martin-Mola, E; De Miguel, E. Increased plasma levels of homocysteine and other thiol compounds in rheumatoid arthritis women. *Clin Biochem*, 1999, 32, 65–70.

[107] Haagsma, CJ; Blom, HJ. Influence of sulphasalazine; methotrexate; and the combination of both on plasma homocysteine concentrations in patients with rheumatoid arthritis; *Ann Rheum Dis.*, 1999, 58, 79–84.

[108] Morgan, SL; Baggott, JE; Lee, JY. Folic acid supplementation prevents deficient blood folate levels and hyperhomocysteinemia during longterm; low dose methotrexate therapy for rheumatoid arthritis: implications for cardiovascular disease prevention. *J Rheumatol.*, 1998, 25, 441–446.

[109] Chiang, EP; Bagley, PJ; Selhub, J; Nadeau, M. Abnormal vitamin B_6 status is associated with severity of symptoms in patients with rheumatoid arthritis. *Am J Med.*, 2003, 114, 283–287.

[110] Lazzerini, PL; Capecchi, S; Bisogno, M; Galeazzi, R. Reduction in plasma homocysteine level in patients with rheumatoid arthritis given pulsed glucocorticoid treatment; Reduction in plasma homocysteine level in patients with rheumatoid arthritis given pulsed glucocorticoid treatment. *Ann Rheum Dis.*, 2003, 62, 694–695.

[111] Knight, BL; Perombelon, YF; Soutar, AK; Wade, DP; Seed, M. Catabolism of lipoprotein(a) in familial hypercholesterolemia subjects. *Atherosclerosis*, 1991, 87, 227-237.

[112] Maeda, S; Abe, A; Seishima, M; Makino, K; Noma, A; Kawade, M. Transient changes of serum lipoprotein(a) as an acute phase protein. *Atherosclerosis*, 1989, 78, 145-150.

[113] Berg, K; Dahlen, G; Frick, MH. Lp(a) lipoprotein and pre-B-lipoprotein in patients with coronary heart disease. *Clin Genet.*, 1974, 230-235.

[114] Rhoads, GG; Dahlen, G; Berg, K; Morton, EN; Dannenberg, AL. Lp(a) lipoprotein as a risk factor of myocardial infarction. *JAMA*, 1986, 256, 2.540.2.544.

[115] Rosengren, A; Wilhelmsen, L; Eriksson, E; Risberg, B; Widel, H. Lipoprotein(a) and coronary heart disease: a prospective case-control study in a population sample of middle aged men. *Br Med J.*, 1990, 301, 1.248-1.251.

[116] Dahlen, GH. Lp(a) lipoprotein in cardiovascular disease; *Atherosclerosis,* 1994, 108, 111–126.

[117] Dursun, D; Harun, E. Lp(a) lipoprotein and lipids in patients with rheumatoid arthritis: serum levels and relationship to inflammation. *Rheumatol Int.*, 2005, 25(4), 241-5.

[118] Kannel, WB; Wolf, OA; Castelli, WP; D'Agostino, RB. Fibrinogen and risk of cardiovascular disease: the Framingham study. *JAMA*, 1987, 258, 1.183-1.186.

[119] Kannel, WB. Factores de riesgo de coronariopatía: actualización del estudio de Framingham. Hospital Practice (ed. esp.), 1991, 6, 45-55.

[120] Stec, JJ; Silbershatz, H; Tofler, GH; Matheney, TH; Sutherland, P; Lipinska, I; et al. Association of fibrinogen with cardiovascular risk factors and cardiovascular disease in the Framingham offspring population. *Circulation*, 2000, 102, 1.634-1.638.

[121] Woodward, M; Lowe, GD; Rumley, A; Tunstall-Pedoe, H. Fibrinogen as a risk factor for coronary heart disease and mortality in middle-aged men and women. The Scottish Heart Health Study. *Eur Heart J.*, 1998, 19(1), 55-62.

[122] Ernst, E; Resch, KL. Fibrinogen as a cardiovascular risk factor: a meta-analysis and review of the literature. *Ann Intern Med*, 1993, 118, 956-963.

[123] Ernst, E. Plasma fibrinogen - an independent cardiovascular risk factor. *J Intern Med*, 1990, 227, 365-372.

[124] Ernst, E. The role of fibrinogen as a cardiovascular risk factor. *Atherosclerosis,* 1993, 100, 1-12.

[125] Heinrich, J; Balleisen, L; Schulte, H; Assmann, G; Van de Loo, J. Fibrinogen and factor VII in the prediction of coronary risk. Results from the PROCAM study in healthy men. *Arterioscler Thromb*, 1994, 14 (1), 54-59.

[126] Danesh, J; Collins, R; Appleby, P; Peto, R. Association of fibrinogen; C-reactive protein; albumin; or leukocyte count with coronary heart disease: meta-analysis of prospective studies. *JAMA*, 1998, 279, 14

[127] Thompson, SG; Kienast, J; Pyke, SDM; Haverkate, F; Van de Loo, JCW. Hemostatic factors and the risk of myocardial infarction or sudden death in patients with angina pectoris. *N Engl J Med.*, 1995, 332, 635-641.

[128] Calvo, A; Monge, N. La microalbuminuria como factor de riesgo cardiovascular. *Semergen*, 2004, 30(3), 110-3.

[129] Roldán, C; Campo, C; Segura, J. Evaluación del riesgo cardiovascular y nuevos factores de arteriosclerosis. *Hipertensión.*, 2005, 22(5), 195-202.

[130] Agrawal, B; Berger, A; Wolf, K; Luft, FC. Microalbuminuria screening by reagent strip predicts cardiovascular risk in hypertension. *J Hypertens.*, 1996, 14, 223-8.

[131] Roest, M; Banga, JD; Janssen, WMT; Grobbee, DE; Sixma, JJ; de Jong, PE; et al. Excessive urinary albumin levels are associated with future cardiovascular mortality in postmenopausal women. *Circulation*, 2001, 103, 3057-61.

[132] Gerstein, HC; Mann, JF; Yi, Q; Zinman, B; Dinneen, SF; Hoogwerf, B; et al. Albuminuria and risk of cardiovascular events; death; and heart failure in diabetic and nondiabetic individuals. *JAMA*, 2001, 286, 421-6.

[133] Hoogeveen, EK; Kostense, PJ; Jager, A; Heine, RJ; Jakobs, C; Bouter LM; et al. Serum Homocysteine level and protein intake are related to risk of microalbuminuria: *The Hoorm Study. Kidney Int.*, 1998, 54, 203-9.

[134] Pedersen, LM; Nordin, H; Svensson, B; et al. Microalbuminuria in patients with rheumatoid arthritis. *Ann Rheum Dis.,* 1995, 54, 189–192.

[135] Maziere, C; Auclair, M; Maziere, JC. Tumor necrosis factor enhances low density lipoprotein oxidative modification by monocytes and endothelial cells. *FEBS Lett*, 1994, 338, 43–46.

[136] Huelmos, A; Battle, E; España, E; López-Bescos, L. Aplicaciones clínicas de la determinación plasmática del péptido natriurético auricular. *Med Intensiva*, 2004, 28(7), 365-375.

[137] Harney, SMJ; Timperley, J; Daly, C; Harin, A. brain natriuretic peptide is a potentially useful screening tool for the detection of cardiovascular disease in patients with rheumatoid arthritis. Lett. 2005.

[138] Fischer, LM; Schlienger, RG; Matter, CM. Discontinuation of nonsteroidal anti-inflammatory drug therapy and risk of acute myocardial infarction. *Arch intern Med.*, 2004, 164, 2472-2476.

[139] Bombardier, C; Laine, L; Reicin, A; Shapiro, D; Burgos-Vargas, R; Davis, B; et al; the VIGOR Study Group. Comparison of upper gastrointestinal toxicity of rofecoxib and naproxen in patients with rheumatoid arthritis. *N Engl J Med*, 2000, 343, 1520-8.

[140] Davis, JM; Maradit-kremers, H. Cumulative glucocorticoid exposure and the risk of cardiovascular events in a population-based cohort of rheumatoid arthritis subjects. *Arthritis Rheum,* 2005, 52, S704.

[141] Boers, M. Influence of glucocorticoids and disease activity on total and high density lipoprotein cholesterol in patients with rheumatoid arthritis. *Ann Rheum Dis,* 2003, 62(9), 842-5.

[142] Hallgren, R; Berne, C; Glucose intolerance in patients with chronic inflammatory diseases is normalized by glucocorticoids. *Acta Med Scand.*, 1983, 213, 351–355.

[143] Svenson, KL; Pollare, T; Lithell, H; Hallgren, R. Impaired glucose handling in active rheumatoid arthritis: relationship to peripheral insulin resistance. *Metabolism*, 1988, 37, 125–130.

[144] Del Rincón, I; O'Leray, DH. Effect of glucorticoids on the arteries in rheumatoid arthritis. *Arthritis and Rheum*, 2004, 50(12), 3813-3822.

[145] Van Halm, VP; Nurmohamed, MT; Twisk, JW. Antirheumatic drugs are associated with reduction of cardiovascular risk in patients with rheumatoid arthritis. *Arthritis Rheum,* 2005, 52.S704.

[146] Wallace, DJ; Linker-Israeli, M; Metzger, AL. The relevance of antimalarial therapy with regard to thrombosis; hypercholesterolemia and cytokines in SLE. *Lupus*, 1993, 2, S13–S15.

[147] Gonzalez-Juanatey, C; Llorca, J; Testa, J. Increased prevalence of severe subclinical atherosclerotic findings in long-term treated rheumatoid arthritis patients without clinically evident atherosclerotic disease; Medicine (Baltimore). 2003, 82, 407–413.

[148] Piercarlo Sarzi-PuttiniTNF-alpha; rheumatoid arthritis; and heart failure: a rheumatological dilemma. *Autoimmun Rev.*, 2005, 4(3), 153-61.

[149] Packer, M; Chung, E; Batra, S; Kereiakes, DJ; Willerson, JT. Randomized placebo-controlled dose-ranging trial of infliximab; a monoclonal antibody to tumor necrosis factor-α; in moderate to severe heart failure Paper presented at: Annual Meeting of the Heart *Failure Society of America*, 2002, Boca Raton; Fla 2002.

[150] Chung, ES; Packer, M; Lo, KH; Fasanmade, AA; Willerson, JT. Anti-TNF Therapy Against Congestive Heart Failure Investigators. Randomized; double-blind; placebo-controlled; pilot trial of infliximab; a chimeric monoclonal antibody to tumor necrosis factor-alpha; in patients with moderate-to-severe heart failure: results of the anti-TNF Therapy Against Congestive Heart Failure (ATTACH) trial; *Circulation*, 2003, 107, 3133–3140.

[151] Grundmann, S; Hoefer, I. Anti-tumor necrosis factor alpha therapies attenuate adaptive arteriogenesis in the rabbit. *Am J Physiol Heart Circ Physiol*, 2005, 289, 1497-1505.

[152] Hurlimann, D; Foster, A. Anti-tumor necrosis alpha treatment improves endothelial function in patients with rheumatoid arthritis. *Circulation*, 2002, 106, 2184-2187.

[153] Jacobsson, LT; Turesson, C. Treatment with tumor necrosis factor blockers is associated with a lower incidence of first cardiovascular events in patients with rheumatoid arthritis. *J Rheumatol,* 2005, 32, 1213-1218.

[154] Gonzalez-Juanatey, C; Testa, A. Active but transient improvement of endotelial function in rheumatoid arthritis patients undergoing long term treatment with anti-tumor necrosis alpha antibody. *Arthritis and Rheum*. 2004, 51, 447-450.

[155] Pérez-Galán, MJ; Salvatierra-Ossorio, J. Influencia del bloqueo del factor de necrosis tumoral alfa (infliximab) en el metabolismo lipídico de pacientes con artritis reumatoide. *Med Clin Barc*, 2006, 126(19), 757-9.

[156] Popa, C; Netea, MG. Influence of anti-tumor necrosis factor therapy on cardiovascular risk factors in patients with active rheumatoid arthritis. *Ann Rheum Dis.,* 2005, 64, 303-305.

[157] Leung, BP; Sattar, N; Crilly, A; Prach, M; McCarey, DW; Payne, H; et al.; A novel anti-inflammatory role for simvastatin in inflammatory arthritis; *J Immunol,* 2003, 170, 1524–1530.

[158] Leung, WH; Wong, CP. Beneficial effect of cholesterol-lowering therapy on coronary endothelium-dependent relaxation in hypercholesterolaemic patients; *Lancet*, 1993, 341, 1496–1500.

[159] Anderson, TJ; Meredith, IT; Yeung, AC. The effect of cholesterol-lowering and antioxidant therapy on endothelium-dependent coronary vasomotion. *N Engl J Med.*, 1995, 332, 488–493.

[160] Perticone, F; Ceravolo, R; Maio, R. Effects of atorvastatin and vitamin C on endothelial function of hypercholesterolemic patients; *Atherosclerosis,* 2000, 152 : 511–518.

[161] Masumoto, A; Hirooka, Y; Hironaga, K. Effect of pravastatin on endothelial function in patients with coronary artery disease (cholesterol-independent effect of pravastatin). *Am J Cardiol.*, 2001, 88, 1291–1294.

[162] McCarey, DW; McInnes, IB; Madhok, R. Trial of Atorvastatin in Rheumatoid Arthritis (TARA), double-blind; randomised placebo-controlled trial. *Lancet*, 2004, 363, 2015–2021.

[163] Van Doornum, S; McColl, G. Atorvastatin reduces arterial stiffness in patients with rheumatoid arthritis. *Ann Rheum Dis.,* 2004, 63, 1572-1575.

[164] Hermann, F; Foster, A. Simvastatin improves endothelial function in patients with rheumatoid arthritis. *J Am Coll Cardiol.*, 2005, 45, 461-464.

[165] Tikiz, C; Utuk, O. Effects of angiotensin-converting enzyme inhibition and statin treatment on inflammatory markets and endothelial functions in patients with longterm threumatoid arthritis. *J Rheumatol,* 2005, 32, 2095-2101.

[166] Wood, D; De Backer, G; Faergeman, O; Graham, I; Mancia, G; Pyorala, K; et al. Prevention of coronary heart disease in clinical practice: Recommendations of the Second Joint Task Force of European and other Societies on Coronary Prevention. *Atherosclerosis,* 1998, 140, 199-270.

[167] Comité español interdisciplinario para la prevención cardiovascular (CEIPC). Adaptación española de la Guía Europea de Prevención Cardiovascular. Clin Invest Arterioscler. 2005, 17(1), 19-33.

[168] International Lipid Information Bureau. The ILIB lipid handbook for clinical practice. Blood lipids and coronary heart disease. 2ª ed. New York: ILIB; 2000.

[169] Expert Panel on Detection; Evaluation; and Treatment of High Blood Cholesterol in Adults. Executive summary of the third report of the National Cholesterol Education Program (NCEP) Expert Panel on Detection; Evaluation; and Treatment of High Blood Cholesterol in Adults (Adult Treatment Panel III). *JAMA.*, 2001, 285, 2486-97.

[170] Wilson, PW; D'Agostino, RB; Levy, D; Belanger, AM; Silvershatz, H; Kannel, WB. Prediction of coronary heart disease using risk factor categories. *Circulation,* 1998, 97, 1837-47.

[171] Stamler, J; Stamler, R; Neaton, JD; Wentworth, D; Daviglus, ML; Garside, D; et al. Low-risk factor profile and long-term cardiovascular and noncardiovascular mortality and life expectancy: findings for 5 large cohorts of young adult and middle-aged men and women. *JAMA*, 1999, 282, 2012-8.

[172] Greenland, P; Abrams, J; Aurigemma, GP; Bond, MG; Clark, LT; Criqui, MH. AHA Conference Proceedings. Prevention Conference V. Beyond secondary prevention: identifying the high-risk patient for primary prevention. Noninvasive tests of atherosclerotic burden. *Circulation,* 2000, 101, E16-22.

[173] Criqui, MH; Denenberg, JO; Langer, RD; Fronek, A. The epidemiology of peripheral arterial disease: importance of identifying the population at risk. *Vasc Med.*, 1997, 2, 221-6.

[174] Zheng, ZJ; Sharrett, AR; Chambless, LE; Rosamond, WD; Nieto, FJ; Sheps, DS; et al. Associations of ankle-brachial index with clinical coronary heart disease; stroke and preclinical carotid and popliteal atherosclerosis: the Atherosclerosis Risk in Communities (ARIC) study. *Atherosclerosis.,* 1997, 131, 115-25.

[175] Murabito, JM; Evans, JC; Nieto, K; Larson, MG; Levy, D; Wilson, PW. Prevalence and clinical correlates of peripheral arterial disease in the Framingham Offspring Study. *Am Heart J.*, 2002, 143, 961-5.

[176] Newman, AB; Siscovick, DS; Manolio, TA; Polak, J; Fried, LP; Borhani, NO; et al. Ankle-arm index as a marker of atherosclerosis in the Cardiovascular Health Study. Cardiovascular Heart Study (CHS) Collaborative Research Group. *Circulation,* 1993, 88, 837-45.

[177] Papamichael, CM; Lekakis, JP; Stamatelopoulos, KS; Papaioannou, TG; Alevizaki, MK; Cimponeriu, AT; et al. Ankle-brachial index as a predictor of the extent of coronary atherosclerosis and cardiovascular events in patients with coronary artery disease. *Am J Cardiol*, 2000, 86, 615-8.

[178] Manzano, L; García-Díaz, JD; Gómez-Cerezo, J. Valor de la determinación del índice tobillo-brazo en pacientes de riesgo vascular sin enfermedad aterotrombótica conocida: estudio VITAMIN. Rev Esp *Cardiol*, 2006, 59(7), 1-9.

[179] Hooi, JD; Stoffers, HE; Kester, AD; Rinkens, PE; Kaiser, V; Van Ree, JW; et al. Risk factors and cardiovascular diseases associated with asymptomatic peripheral arterial occlusive disease. The Limburg PAOD Study. Peripheral Arterial Occlusive Disease. *Scand J Prim Health Care.*, 1998, 16, 177-82.

[180] Allan, PL; Mowbray, PI; Lee, AJ; Fowkes, FG. Relationship between carotid intima-media thickness and symptomatic and asymptomatic peripheral arterial disease. The Edinburgh *Artery Study. Stroke*, 1997, 28, 348-353.

[181] Ogren, M; Hedblad, B; Jungquist, G; Isacsson, SO; Lindell, SE; Janzon, L. Low ankle-brachial pressure index in 68-year-old men: prevalence, risk factors and prognosis. Results from prospective population study Men born in 1914, Malmo, Sweden. *Eur J Vasc Surg.*, 1993, 7, 500-6.

[182] Curb, JD; Masaki, K; Rodríguez, BL; Abbott, RD; Burchfiel, CM; Chen, R; et al. Peripheral artery disease and cardiovascular risk factors in the elderly. The Honolulu Heart Program. *Arterioscler Thromb Vasc Biol.*, 1996, 16, 1495-500.

[183] Shinozaki, T; Hasegawa, T; Yano, E. Ankle-arm index as an indicator of atherosclerosis: its application as a screening method. *J Clin Epidemiol*, 1998, 51, 1263-9.

[184] Newman, AB; Shemanski, L; Manolio, TA; Cushman, M; Mittelmark, M; Polak, JF; et al. Ankle-arm index as a predictor of cardiovascular disease and mortality in the Cardiovascular Health Study. The Cardiovascular Health Study Group. *Arterioscler Thromb Vasc Biol*, 1999, 19, 538-45.

[185] Jager, A; Kostense, PJ; Ruhe, HG; Heine, RJ; Nijpels, G; Dekker, JM; et al. Microalbuminuria and peripheral arterial disease are independent predictors of cardiovascular and all-cause mortality; especially among hypertensive subjects: five-year follow-up of the Hoorn Study. *Arterioscler Thromb Vasc Biol*, 1999, 19, 617-24.

[186] Vogt, MT; McKenna, M; Wolfson, SK; Kuller, LH. The relationship between ankle brachial index; other atherosclerotic disease; diabetes; smoking and mortality in older men and women. *Atherosclerosis,* 1993, 101, 191-202.

[187] Criqui, MH; Langer, RD; Fronek, A; Feigelson, HS; Klauber, MR; McCann, TJ; et al. Mortality over a period of 10 years in patients with peripheral arterial disease. *N Engl J Med*, 1992, 326, 381-6.

[188] Abbott, RD; Rodríguez, BL; Petrovitch, H; Yano, K; Schatz, IJ; Popper, JS; et al. Ankle-brachial blood pressure in elderly men and the risk of stroke: the Honolulu Heart Program. *J Clin Epidemiol*, 2001, 54, 973-8.

[189] Ogren, M; Hedblad, B; Isacsson, SO; Janzon, L; Jungquist, G; Lindell, SE. Ten year cerebrovascular morbidity and mortality in 68 year old men with asymptomatic carotid stenosis. *BMJ.*, 1995, 310, 1294-8.

[190] Tsai, AW; Folsom, AR; Rosamond, WD; Jones, DW. Ankle-brachial index and 7-year ischemic stroke incidence: the ARIC Study. *Stroke.,* 2001, 32, 1721-4.

[191] Lahoz, C; Vicente, I; Taboada, M; Laguna, F; Mostaza, JM. Índice tobillo-brazo y riesgo cardiovascular estimado mediante la función SCORE en sujetos no diabéticos en prevención primaria. *Clin Invest Arterioscl,* 2006, 18, 45-50.

[192] Junyent, M; Gilabert, R. Ecografía carotídea en la evaluación de aterosclerosis preclínica. Distribución de valores del grosor íntima-media y frecuencia de placas de ateroma en una cohorte comunitaria española. *Med Clin(Barc),* 2005, 125(20), 770-4.

[193] O'Leary, DH; Polak, JF; Kronmal, RA; Manolio, TA; Burke, GL; Wolfson, SK; Jr. Carotid-artery intima and media thickness as a risk factor for myocardial infarction and stroke in older adults: Cardiovascular Health Study. *N Engl J Med.*, 1999, 340, 14-22.

[194] Salonen, JT; Salonen, R. Ultrasonographically assessed carotid morphology and the risk of coronary heart disease. *Arterioscler Thromb.*, 1991, 11, 1245-9.

[195] Bots, ML; Hoes, AW; Koudstaal, PJ; Hofman, A; Grobbee, DE. Common carotid intima-media thickness and risk of stroke and myocardial infarction: the Rotterdam Study. *Circulation,* 1997, 96, 1432-7.

[196] Chambless, LE; Heiss, G; Folsom, AR; Rosamond, W; Szklo, M; Sharrett, AR; et al. Association of coronary heart disease incidence with carotid arterial wall thickness and major risk factors: the Atherosclerosis Risk in Communities (ARIC) Study; 1987-1993.*Am J Epidemiol*, 1997, 146, 483-94.

[197] Hodis, HN; Mack, WJ; LaBree, L; Selzer, RH; Liu, CR; Liu, CH; et al. Te role of carotid arterial intima-media thickness in predicting clinical coronary events. *Ann Intern Med.*, 1998, 128, 262-9.

[198] Iglesias del Sol, A; Bots, ML; Grobbee, DE; Hofman, A; Witteman, JCM. Carotid intima-media thickness at different sites: relation to incident myocardial infarction. *Eur Heart J.*, 2002, 23, 934-40.

[199] Chambless, LE; Folsom, AR; Clegg, LX; Sharrett, AR; Shahar, E; Nieto, FJ; et al. Carotid wall thickness is predictive of incident clinical stroke: the Atherosclerosis Risk in Communities (ARIC) Study; 1987-1993. *Am J Epidemiol.*, 2000, 151, 478-87.

[200] Hollander, M; Bots, ML; Iglesias del Sol, A; Koudstaal, PJ; Witteman, JCM; Grobbee, DE; et al. Carotid plaques increase the risk of stroke and subtypes of cerebral infarction in asymptomatic elderly. The Rotterdam Study. *Circulation,* 2002, 105, 2872-7.

[201] Belcaro, G; Nicolaides, AN; Laurora, G; Cesarone, MR; De Sanctis, M; Incandela, L; et al. Ultrasound morphology classification of the arterial wall and cardiovascular events in a 6-year follow-up study. *Arterioscler Thromb Vasc Biol*, 1996, 16, 851-6.

[202] Ebrahim, S; Papacosta, O; Whincup, P; Wannamethee, G; Walker, M; Nicolaides, AN; et al. Carotid plaque; intima-media thickness; cardiovascular risk factors; and prevalent cardiovascular disease in men and women. *The British Regional Heart Study Stroke*, 1999, 30, 841-50.

[203] Bastarrika, G; Pueyo, J. Detección y cuantificación de la calcificación de las arterias coronarias. *Perspectiva radiológica. Radiología*, 2004, 46(1), 1-8.

[204] Margolis, JR; Chen, JT; Kong, Y. The diagnostic and prognostic significance of coronary artery calcification. A report of 800 cases. *Radiology*, 1980, 137, 609-616.

[205] Detrano, RC; Wong, ND. Prognostic significance of cardiac cinepluoroscopy for coronary calcific deposits in asymptomatic high risk subjects. *J Am Coll Cardiol*, 1994, 24, 354-358.

[206] Masuda, Y; Naíto, S. Coronary artery calcification detected by TC: clinical significance and angiographic correlates. *Angiology*, 1990, 41, 1037-1047.

[207] Arad, Y; Spadaro, LA; Goodman, K; Newstein, D; Guerci, AD. Prediction of coronary events with electron beam computed tomography. *J Am Coll Cardiol.*, 2000, 36, 1253-60.

[208] Agatston, AS; Janowitz, WR. Quantification of coronary artery calcium using ultrafast computed tomography. *J Am Coll Cardiol*, 1990, 15, 827-832.

[209] O'Rourke, RA; Brundage, BH. American college of cardiology7 American heart association expert consensus Document on electron beam computed tomography for the diagnosis and prognosis of coronary artery disease. *J Am Coll Cardiol.*, 2000, 36, 326-340.

[210] Callister, TQ; Raggi, P; Croil, B. Effect of HMG-CoA reductase inhibitors on coronary artery disease and assessed by electron beam computed tomography. *N Engl J Med.*, 1998, 339, 1972-1978.

[211] Zambón, D; Gilabert, R; Ros, E. Aterosclerosis carotídea evaluada por ecografía bidimensional en pacientes con hipercolesterolemia primaria. Med Clin (Barc). 1995, 105, 761-7.

[212] Rumberger, JA; Sheedy, PF; Breen, JF. Electrom bean computed tomography and coronary artery disease: scanning for coronary artery calcification. *Mayo Clin Proc.*, 1996, 71, 369-377.

[213] O'Rourke, RA; Brundage, BH; Froelicher, VG. American College of Cardiology/ American Heart Association expert consensus document on electron-beam computed tomography for the diagnosis and prognosis of coronary artery disease. *Circulation,* 2000, 102, 126-40.

[214] Del Rincon, I. Lower limb arterial incompressibility and obstruction in rheumatoid arthritis. *Ann Rheum Dis.,* 2005, 64(3), 425-32.

[215] Alkaabi, JK; Ho, M; Levison, R. Rheumatoid arthritis and macrovascular disease. *Rheumatology*, 2003, 42, 292-297.

[216] Petri, M; Hamper, U. Frequency of atherosclerosis detected by carotid duplex in systemic lupus srythematosus. *Arthritis Rheum,* 1997, 40 (Suppl), 219.

[217] Roman, MJ; Salmon, J; Sobel, R. Premature athrosclerosis and myocardial hypertrophy in SLE and antiphospholipid antibody syndrome. *Arthritis Rheum,* 1997, 40, S302.

[218] Levenson, J; Giral, P; Razavian, M; Garipey, J; Simon, A. Fibrinogen and silent atherosclerosis in subjects with cardiovascular risk factors. *Atheroscler Thromb Vasc Biol*, 1995, 15, 1263-8.

[219] Falaschi, F; Ravelli, A; Martignoli, A; Migliavacca, D; Sartori, M; Pistorio, A; et al. Nephrotic-range proteinuria; the major risk factor for early atheroscleosis in juvenile-onset systemic lupus erythematosus. *Arthritis Rheum,* 2000, 43, 1405-9.

[220] Roman, MJ; Salmon, JE; Sobel, R; Lockshin, MD; Sammaritano, L; Schwartz, JE; et al. Prevalence and relation to risk factors of carotid atherosclerosis and left ventricular hypertrophy in systemic lupus erythematosus and antiphpholipid antibody syndrome. *Am J Cardiology*, 2001, 87, 663-6.

[221] Svenungsson, E; Jensen-Urstad, K; Heimbürger, M; Silveira, A; Hamsten, A; de Faire, U; et al. Risk factors for cardiovascular disease in systemic lupus erythematosus. *Circulation*, 2001, 16, 1887-93.

[222] Roman, MJ. Prevalence and Correlates of Accelerated Atherosclerosis in Systemic Lupus Erythematosus. *N Engl J Med,* 2003, 349(25), 2399-2403.

[223] Beltrán, J. Aterosclerosis subclínica en la artritis reumatoide. Técnicas no invasivas de detección. *Semin Fund Esp Reumatol*, 2005, 6, 64-71.

[224] González-Juanatey, C; Llorca, J; Testa, A; Revuelta, J. Increased prevalence of severe subclinical atherosclerotis findings in long-term treated rheumatoid arthritis patients without clinically evident atherosclerotic disease. *Medicine (Baltimore).,* 2003, 82, 407-413.

[225] Kumeda, Y; Inaba, M; Goto, H; Nagata, M. Increased thickness of the arterial intima-media detected by ultrasonography in patients with rheumatoid arthritis. *Arthritis Rheum,* 2002, 46, 1489-14997.

[226] Young-Beom, P; Chul-Woo, A; Hyon, KC. Atherosclerosis in rheumatoid arthritis. Morphologic evidence obtained by carotid ultrasound. *Arthritis Rheum,* 2002, 46, 1714-1719.

[227] Roman, MJ; Devereux, RB; Schwartz, JE. Arterial stiffness in chronic inflammatory diseases. *Hypertension,* 2005, 46, 194-199.

[228] Del Rincón, I; Williams, K. Association between carotid atherosclerosis and markers of inflammation in rheumatoid arthritis patients and healthy subjects. *Arthritis Rheum,* 2003, 48, 1833-1840.

[229] Del Rincón, I; Freeman, G; Haas, R. Relative contribution of cardiovascular risk factors and rheumatoid arthritis clinical manifestations to atherosclerosis. *Arthritis Rheum,* 2005, 52, 3413-3423.

[230] Abu-Shakra, M; Polychuck, I; Szendro, G. Duplex study of the carotid and femoral arteries of patients with rheumatoid arthritis: a controlled study. Seminars in *Arthritis Rheum,* 2005, 35, 18-23.

[231] Roman, MJ; Moeller, E. Preclinical carotid atherosclerosis in patients with rheumatoid arthritis. *Ann Intern Med*, 2006, 144(4).249-256.

[232] Maheer, JE; Bielak, LF; Raz, JA; Sheedy, PF; Schwartz, RS; Peyser, PA. Progresion of coronary artery calcification: a pilot study. *Mayo Clin Proc*, 1999, 74, 347-55.

[233] Asanuma, Y. Premature Coronary-Artery Atherosclerosis in Systemic Lupus Erythematosus. *N Engl J Med*, 2003, 349(25), 2407-14.

[234] Chung, C; Oeser, A; Raggi, P. Increased coronary-artery atherosclerosis in rheumatoid arthritis: relationship to disease duration and cardiovascular risk factors. *Arthritis Rheum*, 2005, 52(10), 3045-53.

[235] Goldeli, O; Dursun, E. Dispersión of ventricular repolarization: a new marker of ventricular arrhythmias in patients with rheumatoid artritis. *J Rheumatol*, 1998, 25, 447-50.

[236] Cindas, A; Gökce-Kutsal, Y. QT dispersión and cardiac involvement in patients with rheumatoid arthritis. Scand *J Rheumatol*, 2002, 31, 22-6.

[237] Tlustochowicz, W; Piotrowicz, R. 24-h ECG monitoring in patients with rheumatoid arthritis. *Eur Heart J*, 1995, 16(6), 848-51.

[238] Freire, M; Graña, J; Atanes, A. Artritis reumatoide. Guías clínicas del Servicio Gallego de Salud (SERGAS). 2004, 4(39).

[239] Lindner, UK; Dubin, DB. Introducción a la electrocardiografía. Ed. Springer-Verlag Ibérica; 6ª edición; p 435.

[240] Hiat, WR. Medical treatment of peripheral disease and claudication. N *Engl J Med*, 2001, 344, 1608-21.

[241] Fernández-Miranda, C; Aranda, JL; Paz, M. Aterosclerosis subclínica de la arteria carótida en pacientes con enfermedad coronaria. *Med Clin (Barc).*, 2001, 116, 441-6.

[242] Belcaro, G; Renton, S. Ultrasonic biopsy-A non-invasive screening tecnique to evaluate the cardiovascular risk and to follow up the progresión and the regresión of arteriosclerosis. *Vasa*, 1991, 20, 40-50.

[243] Callister, TQ; Bruce, C. Coronary artery disease: improved reproducibility of calcium scoring with an electrom-bean CT volumetric method. *Radiology*, 1998, 208, 807-814.

[244] Carmona, L; Ballina, J. EPISER Study Group. The burden of musculoskeletal diseases in the general population of Spain: results from a national survey. *Ann Rheum Dis.*, 2001, 60, 1040-1045.

[245] Emery, P; Breedveld, FC; Jubb, RW. Efficacy and safety of leflunomide vs methotrexate in rheumatoid arthritis. Results of double-blind randomized; 2 year trial. *Arthritis Rheum.*, 1999, 42, S271, 1203

In: Rheumatoid Arthritis: Prevalence, Risk...
Editor: Michael H. Madsen
ISBN: 978-1-61761-931-1

Chapter 2

A Review on Neurobiomechanical Changes in Rheumatoid Arthritis

Aparna Rajagopalan
School of Medical Sciences, Sydney Medical School,
University of Sydney, Lidcombe, NSW, Australia

1.1. Rheumatoid Arthritis- A General Perspective

Rheumatoid Arthritis (RA) is a chronic, inflammatory, incurable disorder of uncertain etiology, associated with significant morbidity. It is a systemic autoimmune disorder characterized by symmetric inflammation of synovial joints leading to progressive erosion of cartilage and bone. Patients require potentially lifelong treatment and there may be a substantial socio-economic impact (Siddiqui, 2007). Generally, the onset of RA is seen in middle age (40–70 years), with a 2.5- fold higher prevalence in women than in men (Lee & Weinblatt, 2001). Genetic polymorphisms of the major histocompatibility complex (MHC) II have been implicated in a predisposition to RA in various ethnic groups. The clinical criteria for RA has been extensively reviewed (Arnett *et al.*, 1988a).

Joint stiffness is the cardinal clinical symptom of RA, which frequently affects the upper limb, rendering the affected limb disabled. The known pathophysiology of RA affected joint includes inflammation which produces numerous chemical mediators resulting in central sensitization causing hyperalgesia. But the nature and cause of the stiffness need to be elucidated. For this to be studied, the underlying pathophysiology and the current understanding need to be reviewed.

1.2. Pathophysiology

The etiology of RA is thought to be related to multiple genetic and exogenous factors. The synovium, the connective tissue membrane that lines the joint is the primary site of pathology in RA. Although the processes that maintain long-term inflammation of the synovium in RA have been well studied (Zvaifler, 1973), those initiating the inflammation have not been established. The synovium becomes inflamed resulting in joint swelling and joint destruction as the immune system attacks the tissues lining the joints.

Arthritis usually involves some form of damage to, or destruction of joint parts. In the case of RA, the synovial membrane becomes inflamed. The membrane becomes thick and stiff. Inflammation causes proliferation of fibroblasts that changes the characteristics of the membrane in a short period of time (Curtiss, 1964). The fibrosis and the vasculitis of the synovial membrane subsequently leads to the damage of articular cartilages, an important tissue for joint function (Mills, 1970). The membrane is also attacked by white blood cells, which can damage or kill tissue in the joint.

1.3. Symptoms

All forms of arthritis share certain symptoms in common. These symptoms include pain, swelling, and stiffness in the joint (Arnett *et al.*, 1988a). These symptoms may develop slowly over time or they may begin quite suddenly. After a period of time, joints may actually become deformed. Patients may find it difficult to straighten their fingers and toes, or their hands and feet may curve outward in an abnormal way. As the condition progresses, the muscles around the joint waste away, the cartilage in the joint and the bone underneath erode away, and eventually the whole joint is filled with fibrous scar tissue until it freezes completely.

Early diagnosis and treatment is an integral part of the management of RA, with the aims of reducing and controlling symptoms of joint pain and inflammation, minimizing loss of function, and reducing joint damage and disability (Guidelines for the management of rheumatoid arthritis: 2002 update). Since RA is an inflammatory condition, first-line therapy has traditionally included medications that suppress inflammation, such as nonsteroidal anti-inflammatory drugs (NSAIDs) and glucocorticoids to reduce inflammation, therefore pain and swelling (Gaffo *et al.*, 2006). Disease-modifying antirheumatic drugs (DMARDs), such as methotrexate, have long been the mainstay of treatment and are still advocated as a first-line option in newly diagnosed patients with RA (Luqmani *et al.*, 2006). However, based on emerging research (Feldmann *et al.*, 1996; Moreland, 1999; Choy & Panayi, 2001) on the roles of inflammatory mediators in the pathogenesis of RA, therapies targeted at the different aspects of the inflammatory cascade, most notably TNF-α, IL-1, IL-6, T-cell signaling cells, and B-cells, have been developed (Doan & Massarotti, 2005; Goldblatt & Isenberg, 2005; Smolen *et al.*, 2007).

1.4. Factors Contributing to Functional Loss in Arthritis

Functional disability in terms of mobility and a wide range of upper limb tasks are the long term result of RA. A subjective complaint of localized or generalized loss of mobility of the joints, with or without pain, is reported by patients especially in the morning (Lineker *et al.*, 1999). The factors that have been observed to contribute to this condition include joint stiffness, pain, reduced range of motion and muscle weakness associated with muscle wasting (Ekdahl *et al.*, 1989). It is thus evident that the disability is mediated by a complex pattern of sensorimotor changes secondary to the joint disease.

These underlying neuromuscular mechanisms have received little attention in the research literature, though they are involved in producing disability, and are poorly understood. Increased resistance to joint movement in RA may be due to centrally mediated neural factors and/or peripheral mechanical factors. The articular manifestations of RA such as inflammation are well established. However, the extra-articular factors such as muscle factors and neural factors are less studied. There is very limited clinical documentation of motor disability in RA and the diagnostic criteria do not include a motor scale or performance rating.

1.4.1. Muscle Function in Joint Disorders

Muscle weakness and atrophy are frequently observed in knee joint disorders. This has been studied in osteoarthritis (OA) of the knee (Wessel, 1996; Slemenda *et al.*, 1997; O'Reilly *et al.*, 1998), where reduced knee extensor muscle strength and volume have been found compared to healthy people. Decreased quadriceps strength has been shown to be related to the presence of OA in the knee (Hassan *et al.*, 2001; Hassan *et al.*, 2002). The same was found in patients with knee ligament injuries (Halkjaer-Kristensen & Ingemann-Hansen, 1985). Muscle fibre atrophy of the quadriceps muscle was observed in knee joint disorders (Nakamura *et al.*, 1986). This is probably caused partially by knee joint pain and inactivity. However, weakness in knee extensors in persons with OA without pain has been reported (Slemenda *et al.*, 1997). The effect of unloading on skeletal muscles has been studied in healthy persons. In one study on healthy subjects, strength, cross-sectional area and muscle biopsies were analyzed in the quadriceps muscle after six weeks of bed rest (Berg *et al.*, 1997). The study reported that the knee extensor torque was reduced by 25%, cross-sectional muscle area was reduced by 14% and muscle fibre cross-sectional area was reduced by 18%.

The effect of artificially induced knee effusion on muscle strength has also been studied experimentally in healthy subjects. Both reduction of knee extensor strength and inhibition of reflex-evoked muscle contraction were found (Deandrade *et al.*, 1965b; Kennedy *et al.*, 1982). A relationship between the degree of knee effusion and reduction in knee extensor muscle strength has also been found in chronic knee arthritis. It was observed that progressive inhibition occurred in knee extensor torque when the intra-articular volume and pressure increased (Geborek *et al.*, 1989). Joint aspiration of knee effusion immediately increased quadriceps muscle strength (Fahrer *et al.*, 1988). This arthrogenous muscle weakness is apparently caused by reflex inhibition, since it is partly dependent on afferent stimuli from the joint (Stokes & Young, 1984). Experimental studies in rats have shown rapid muscle atrophy one week after artificially induced arthritis (Herbison *et al.*, 1979). Therefore, there is a possibility that the joint effusion, caused by inflammation could be a potential source of reflex inhibition in RA patients.

1.4.2. Joint Distension and Muscle Weakness

Joint injury inhibits voluntary contraction of muscles acting across the joint and leads to muscle wasting (Iles *et al.*, 1990). It is also well established that knee joint effusion, whether acute (Shakespeare, 1985), chronic (Fahrer *et al.*, 1988), or experimentally induced (deAndrade *et al.*, 1965a; Hopkins *et al.*, 2001; Hopkins *et al.*, 2002), results in weakness and wasting of the quadriceps musculature. This phenomenon has been termed *arthrogenic muscle inhibition* (AMI) (Hopkins & Ingersoll, 2000).

1.4.3. Arthrogenic Muscle Inhibition

AMI is a pre-synaptic, ongoing reflex inhibition of musculature surrounding a joint following distension or damage to structures of that joint. AMI is a natural response designed to protect the joint from further damage (Hopkins & Ingersoll, 2000) (Ingersoll *et al.*, 2003). Pain and disuse are hypothesized to be the reason for the inhibition and muscle atrophy following joint injury (Helliwell & Jackson, 1994). However, studies have shown that AMI can occur independently of the pain sensation (Shakespeare, 1985; Young, 1993). AMI has been identified in subjects with both symptomatic and asymptomatic OA (Arokoski *et al.*, 2002). Even though AMI can occur independently of the conscious appreciation of pain, there is a distinct possibility that afferent impulses from nociceptors may be an important contributing factor (Young, 1993).

Other studies have implied the role of mechanoreceptors in the development of AMI (Hopkins & Ingersoll, 2000). Due to the observation that damage to the joint receptors results in impairment of proprioception and that the extensor musculature of the upper thigh is reduced following knee trauma (to an extent which exceeds inactivity atrophy), the joint receptors have been assigned great importance in AMI (Friewald *et al.*, 1999). AMI therefore results from the activity of many different mechanoreceptors within a joint, namely: Ruffini endings, Golgi-like endings and Pacinian corpuscles (Hopkins & Ingersoll, 2000) and free nerve endings have been observed to play a role in AMI (Friewald *et al.*, 1999; Ingersoll *et al.*, 2003). It has been further hypothesized that chronic mechano-receptor activity surrounding the damaged joint results in the replacement of normal pattern of muscle activity with an adapted functional motor program (Ingersoll *et al.*, 2003).

In animals the wasting caused by experimental arthritis does not occur after interruption of the dorsal roots and therefore seems to require input from receptors in or around the injured joint (Stokes & Young, 1984). Experiments performed on animals have shown that distension of the joint capsule excites slowly adapting receptors, Ruffini endings (Eklund & Skoglund, 1960; Ferrell, 1980). Iles, *et al.*, studied the effect of knee joint distension on quadriceps muscles. They observed that the inhibitory reflex pathway to be active during voluntary contraction. This prompted them to suggest that the inhibition of voluntary contraction following pathological knee joint effusion as simple inhibitory reflex action from afferents activated by joint distension on to quadriceps motoneurons (Iles *et al.*, 1990).

Joint movement provides supraspinal centres with information about the environment and position of that joint. Changes in afferent input to the spinal cord from the joint appear to be the most influential factor associated with AMI (Hopkins & Ingersoll, 2000). Abnormal afferent information from mechano- and nociceptors surrounding the damaged joint, act on inhibitory interneurons, which synapse on the motor neuron (MN) pool of the joint musculature across that joint (Hurley & Newham, 1993). The information from inhibitory interneurons decreases the ability of recruitment within the MN pool, and therefore decreases the force of any contraction stemming from that MN pool (Hurley & Newham, 1993; Hopkins & Ingersoll, 2000). Lesions to peripheral mechanoreceptors could functionally modify central somatosensory pathways. The cortex is involved in complex spatial integration of articular proprioceptive inputs. Measurable changes in muscle strength and muscle atrophy may be due to altered central nervous system under-activation of the involved musculature (Friewald *et al.*, 1999).

Animal studies indicate that the inhibitory action of joint afferents on quadriceps MNs may act at least in part through the Ib inhibitory pathway and cutaneous afferents (Lundberg *et al.*, 1978). Since many joint afferents become active towards the extremes of joint movement (Ferrell, 1980) and Ib afferents are excited by muscle contraction, this convergence may serve to brake an active movement as it reaches its end-point (Iles *et al.*, 1990). It has also been suggested that under normal circumstances, the descending systems that control this pathway may ensure that movement is not inhibited in the mid-range (Lundberg *et al.*, 1978). However, during pathological joint conditions, the braking system might be activated earlier and it could also be more powerful.

Observations by Hopkins *et al.*, suggest that, AMI is likely a combination of pre-synaptic and post-synaptic inhibition. Afferent supply to the interneuron is mediated by post-synaptic neurotransmitters. The information traveling from the interneuron to the MN pool is then pre-synaptically mediated. Reciprocal inhibition is caused by Ia inhibitory interneuron activity. Muscle spindle primary fibres respond to stretch, resulting in afferent activity that synapses on interneurons (one of these interneurons is the Ia inhibitory interneuron). Stimulation of this neuron results in inhibition of the antagonist muscle and its synergists. Also involved in this loop is the γ- MN system. This system is important in functional regulation of Ia receptors in the muscle during contraction. Stimulation of γ- MNs by joint afferents might also contribute to continuous inhibition (Hopkins & Ingersoll, 2000).

1.4.4. Muscle Function in Rheumatoid Arthritis

Reduced strength and muscle volume are known to occur in RA. This is most obvious in muscles near an inflamed joint (Danneskiold-Samsoe & Grimby, 1986a; Hsieh *et al.*, 1987; Ekdahl & Broman, 1992a; Hakkinen *et al.*, 1995). The mechanisms are probably the same as for other joint disorders as discussed above. The muscles of the forearm were studied and reduced grip strength and a reduction in forearm muscle bulk were observed, though muscle wasting was small compared to the reduction in strength (Helliwell & Jackson, 1994). Inactivity due to the disease can lead to a generalized reduction in muscle volume and strength. This is often obvious in patients with severe polyarthritis. Inflammation of the muscles, i.e. polymyositis and/or dermatomyositis, is known to occur as a complication in RA (Brooke & Kaplan, 1972; Halla *et al.*, 1984; Miro *et al.*, 1996). In muscle biopsies there are signs of inflammation and muscle fibre degeneration.

Changes in muscles are also known to occur as a complication with medicines used in RA, e.g. corticosteroids, chloroquine and d-penicillamine. Complications from the nervous system are known to occur in RA and may have affect muscle function. Studies have shown the presence of vasculitic neuropathy, distal symmetric neuropathy and compression neuropathy in some cases of adult RA (Lang *et al.*, 1981; Lanzillo *et al.*, 1998; Sivri & Guler-Uysal, 1998; Bekkelund *et al.*, 1999). Some authors have tried to relate the muscle weakness to functional capacity (Danneskiold-Samsoe & Grimby, 1986b; Ekdahl, 1990; Stucki *et al.*, 1998). A significant correlation between muscle strength and activities of daily living in RA patients has been reported in the literature (Hsieh *et al.*, 1987; Ekdahl & Broman, 1992b; Helliwell & Jackson, 1994; Lindehammar & Lindvall, 2004).

1.4.5. Joint Stiffness as a Contributor to Disability in Arthritis

Although joint stiffness was listed as the cardinal diagnostic symptom of RA (Arnett *et al.*, 1988a) and is used as a clinical indicator of the disease activity, the nature and cause of the stiffness remains unclear. The term 'stiffness' when used in the context of arthritis has done little to clarify the underlying condition. The increased stiffness may be the result of nociceptive feedback-induced changes to the centrally mediated neural factors or local, peripheral changes in the mechanical properties of the muscles.

Objective joint stiffness (OJS) has been defined as the measurable resistance to passive movement when the joint is put through a normal range of motion in the usual functional plane (Thompson *et al.*, 1978). Using biomechanical analysis methods, it is possible to extract and quantify the major components of objective mechanical stiffness, namely, the elastic, viscous and inertial components, and even to estimate the plastic properties of these components (Wright & Johns, 1960b). This data is not available in RA- affected joints and would provide a more complete picture of changes in joint stiffness and the contributing factors. Such measures also have the potential to provide disease markers of improved sensitivity and reliability.

The available literature suggests that changes in OJS do not fully describe the mechanisms leading to functional disability. Haigh, *et al.*, (2003) proposed that the common clinical complaint of subjective rigidity and immobility be described as 'perceived joint stiffness' (PJS), since existing measures of OJS do not correlate well with subjective experience (Helliwell *et al.*, 1988). A further significant limitation of past studies is that the measures were made only in the passive state i.e while the muscles were relaxed. However, patient perception of stiffness arises during maintained isometric contractions and functional tasks.

Stiffness as an input-output property can be measured only with the imposition of a displacement. The stiffness properties measured using different types of displacements and tasks however have been found to vary qualitatively (Kirsch *et al.*, 1994a). Transient perturbations evoke rather complex behaviours (Rack & Westbury, 1974; Nichols & Houk, 1976; Hoffer & Andreassen, 1981; Carter *et al.*, 1990). Continuous sinusoidal displacement has revealed quite a linear behaviour for various joints (Agarwal & Gottlieb, 1977; Brown *et al.*, 1982), with mainly elastic responses with a small viscous component.

When limbs resist sudden displacement, the mass of the limb presents an inertial resistance to the displacement; the muscles offer a 'visco-elastic' resistance to lengthening while reflex muscle contraction opposes the movement. It is difficult to empirically separate and measure the resistive torque that develops in these ways. Previous studies have shown that the resistance of muscles to lengthening and the intensity of reflex activity increases with increasing force of contraction (Marsden *et al.*, 1972; Rack, 1981).

It has been hypothesized that the stiffness observed during movement is different from that observed during posture (Mah, 2001). Under static conditions, resistive torques about a joint varies as a function of muscle length (Gottlieb & Agarwal, 1979; Weiss *et al.*, 1986) and activation (Weiss *et al.*, 1988). The resistive torques that are dependent on the physiological state of muscles are altered during voluntary movement, while the mass and inertia of the limb do not change significantly. Velocity dependency of muscle force may play a significant role in determining the mechanical behaviour of a joint (Milner, 1993). Periarticular structures such as joint capsule, connective tissue, tendons and skin might contribute to joint stiffness.

Increased resistance to passive movement is possibly due to a phenomenon in the muscle called "thixotropy". Warming-up procedures such as stretching of limbs can reduce joint stiffness and increase joint range of motion (Harvey *et al.*, 2002; LaRoche & Connolly, 2006). Such stiffness gradually increases with inactivity or rest. Therefore, it can be stated that the magnitude of the passive opposing load for a voluntary movement depends on the status of the muscles in the preceding time period. As a consequence of motor control mechanisms, the manifestation of such history-dependant variations to skeletal muscle resistance influences voluntary movements. Contribution of thixotropic effects to muscle and joint stiffness remains largely unexplored and this may be because of the theoretical view which equates relaxed muscles to springs (Rack & Westbury, 1974).

1.4.6. Pain as a Contributor to Disability In RA

Many studies have shown that chronic or tonic painful stimuli may alter mechanoreceptor response to mechanical stimuli (Amir & Devor, 2000; Wendler *et al.*, 2001; Kleinbohl *et al.*, 2006). Similarly in RA, chronic pain may alter the threshold for the articular mechanoreceptor thus permitting the transmission of misleading information (Helliwell, 1994). There is evidence to support the theory that there is an expansion of nociceptive receptive fields due to administration of repetitive painful stimulation (Andersen *et al.*, 1994; Arendt-Nielson *et al.*, 1996; Andersen *et al.*, 2001; Andersen *et al.*, 2004; Andersen *et al.*, 2005b).

RA patients report high levels of subjective discomfort (painful sensations) associated with both upper limb tasks and lower limb mobility (Fries *et al.*, 1980). This raises the possibility of the contribution of nociceptive feedback as a limitation to functional ability. Increased nociceptive activity secondary to joint disease could reduce mobility through acute and chronic spinal (reflex) and/or supraspinal mechanisms. A chronic loss of mobility will ultimately lead to disuse atrophy and muscle weakness. Muscle involvement in the pathology of RA has been studied using muscle biopsy. Disuse (Agrawal *et al.*, 2003) and denervation atrophy (Magyar *et al.*, 1977) of type I and type II fibres have been reported in RA previously, based on histopathological studies. These studies have demonstrated the presence of foci of inflammatory cells in the peripheral nerves and in the muscles. These could be significant reasons for pathogenesis following inflammation and the major contributors to muscle wasting. A nerve conduction study however supports hypothesis of disuse atrophy rather than denervation atrophy (Amick, 2005). Further elucidation of the physiological aspects of muscle involvement is needed.

A wide range of neurophysiological techniques is available to test the central or reflex effects of afferent fibre activity. The techniques can reveal changes in the peripheral and central mechanisms mediating the afferent response. The cutaneomuscular reflex (CMR) has been shown to produce powerful inhibition of voluntary muscle activity (Caccia *et al.*, 1973; Jenner & Stephens, 1982; McMahon & Koltzenburg, 1990; Price, 2002). These pathways could thus mediate or contribute to the functional weakness that accompanies RA. Electrical stimulation of cutaneous afferents demonstrates clear phases of excitatory and inhibitory muscle response that can be related to excitatory and inhibitory spinal reflex (and possibly supraspinal) mechanisms.

1.5. Current Methods for Assessment of Functional Disability in RA

1.5.1. Components of Joint Stiffness

Not only is there a need for objective quantification of joint stiffness but stiffness measures have to be analyzed in order to derive individual stiffness components from the total stiffness.

Muscles at rest possess a resting tension. There is no net EMG in the muscles, yet there is a resistance to imposed joint movement (Joyce *et al.*, 1974). Total joint stiffness is composed of an intrinsic (non-reflex) component arising from the mechanical properties of the joint, passive tissue, and active muscle fibres, and a reflex component arising from changes in muscle activation due to sensory responses to stretch. When muscle length changes, there is a passive stiffness to the muscle, which opposes voluntary contraction or imposed movements. This passive stiffness is due to the mechanical properties of the joint and the muscles about the joint.

The mechanical joint stiffness is due to the mass of the limb (due to inertia) and the stiffness due to the tissue themselves. The tissue stiffness can be subdivided into active and passive stiffness. Passive factors include elasticity of the muscle and viscosity of the articular tissue. Active stiffness is due to the electrical activity of the muscle contributed by both voluntary contraction and reflex (Figure 1). This stiffness increases with the increasing number of active crossbridges of actin-myosin. The magnitude of the stiffness can be determined by the amplitude of reflex and neural input to the muscle (Sinkjaer & Hayashi, 1989).

Passive stiffness has two components namely, elasticity and viscosity. Elastic stiffness is a function of displacement and is related to the muscle length (Walsh, 1992a). Viscosity is the function of velocity and mainly due to frictional forces (Joyce *et al.*, 1974; Sinkjaer & Hayashi, 1989). The inertial component is a function of acceleration and is mainly dependent on the mass of the moving joint. Active stiffness is produced by voluntary and involuntary muscle activity.

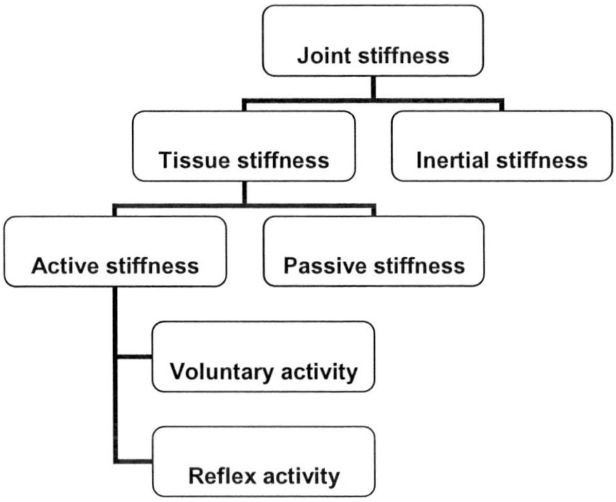

Figure 1. Flow chart shows the components of the total stiffness about a joint

Muscle contraction produces a resistance to the joint movement by formation of crossbridges between actin and myosin (Sinkjaer & Hayashi, 1989). Weak but 'long-lasting' bonds between actin and myosin filaments are spontaneously formed within the sarcomeres under resting conditions (Hill, 1968). Force generation in muscle is a result of the cyclic interaction between myosin heads (crossbridges) and actin in the sarcomere (Brenner & Yu, 1993). Formation of stable crossbridges in a relaxed muscle implies that the muscle fibres are held at a particular length and imposed forces that detach the crossbridges release the muscle fibres from the held length.

Dynamic stiffness describes the relation between changes in joint position and the resulting changes in torque. This stiffness can be separated into its reflex and non-reflex components (Mirbagheri *et al.*, 2000). The reflex stiffness component is due to changes in the level of muscle activation that arise from the afferent response to muscle stretch. The non-reflex or intrinsic stiffness component is due to the mechanical properties of the joint, passive tissue, and active muscle fibres (Sinkjaer *et al.*, 1993). It was found to be difficult to separate the mechanical consequences of reflex activity from those due to passive tissues and active muscles. Different methods were used in various studies to separate the two components of the stiffness. Each method tended to give a different result.

1.5.2. Joint Stiffness in RA

A distinguishing feature of RA is the presence of stiffness, particularly in the morning. Morning stiffness heads the list of diagnostic criteria for RA proposed by the American Rheumatism Association (Arnett *et al.*, 1988a). Subjectively, stiffness is described as a feeling of resistance to movement, slowness in moving the joint in the morning or staying in one position too long (Hazes *et al.*, 1993; Helliwell, 1995). Objectively, stiffness is defined as the measurable resistance to passive motion within a normal range and plane of function (Haigh *et al.*, 2003).

For a long time rheumatoid activity was measured using subjective feeling, observable limitation of range of motion and grip strength (Wright & Johns, 1960b). Objective measures of disability are needed as they can provide information on changes in the status of the patient under treatment (Backlund & Tiselius, 1967). Most current measures focus on muscle strength, not stiffness. Goniometry was a popular method to measure the range of motion. Patient and/or the examiner bias, due to various types of goniometers used (short- and long-armed) and the inconsistencies in the measurement procedures introduced by different examiners (Menadue *et al.*, 2006; Roush *et al.*, 2008), may contaminate this method.

Stiffness is defined by measurable parameters that obey laws of physics, some of which are elasticity, viscosity, friction and inertia. But *in vivo* measurement of stiffness in diseased joint using appropriate devices has proved to be unsuccessful. Early stiffness studies have used arthrographs to measure passive joint stiffness. Arthrograph is a device that has been used commonly to measure passive resistance of a joint to imposed motion. The measurement attempts to define the rheological properties of the tissues in and around the joint (Helliwell *et al.*, 1987a).

Various methods have been used to quantitate stiffness in arthritic joint. Wright (1959), measured grip strength throughout the day, finding marked weakness in the morning and concluded that the patients experienced stiffness when the grip strength was low. Diurnal variation in stiffness was observed in a study, which measured stiffness using an extension spring (Scot, 1960). The changes in the active state of muscle have not been taken into consideration in these studies and there is also no age/sex matched control data to compare the results with.

A method was described that could measure joint stiffness in precise physical terms (Wright & Johns, 1960b). A pendulum driven arthrograph was used to displace the second MCP joint in a sinusoidal manner. The resulting resistive torque was plotted in relation to angular displacement. The torque data was then decomposed into elastic, viscous, plastic and frictional components of stiffness, based on the slope of the torque-angle curves. According to the study, the major component of joint stiffness was plastic stiffness (described by stretch relaxation and creep properties), while the other components had minimal contribution to overall stiffness. These authors also attributed part of the stiffness to the stretching of muscles and tendons about the joint. The arthrograph measurement did not make any correction for the equilibrium position of the joint. The methodology did not include any measurement of muscle activity and the status of the muscle during the experiment was not made explicit.

Backlund *et al.*, (1967) compared subjective and objective stiffness in healthy subjects and patients suffering from RA. Using the pinch test, grip strength measurement and physiological measurement of stiffness of MCP joint, they showed decreasing stiffness and increasing muscle power throughout the day. They hypothesized that the joint capsule also contributed to total stiffness, however the stiffness was not broken down to its components. The methodology indicates the range in which the joint was rotated to be 30° on either side.

Later, horizontally driven knee arthrographs were designed to overcome the mass of the limb (Thompson *et al.*, 1978). The sum of mid-position torques was taken as the measure of elastic stiffness, while the sum of the areas of the individual hysteresis loops served as the measure of viscous stiffness. The authors reported a decrease in measured stiffness in RA patients compared to the control subjects. A similar set-up was devised for a finger arthrograph, which moved the index finger horizontally in flexion-extension plane driven by an electrical motor (Unsworth *et al.*, 1981). Measurements were taken in relation to the equilibrium position of the joint. Sinusoidal displacements were imposed over a 50° range of movement. These investigators also reported no significant increase in the objective stiffness in RA patients compared to normal subjects.

An anthropometric study on the range of motion of fingers in normal subjects indicate that the range of motion of the index finger to be 70.83° $\pm$ 11.09° (Becker & Thakor, 1988). There is a distinct possibility that the large range of displacement caused breakage of the acto-myosin crossbridges, therefore the observed result. There was no EMG recording to show the status of the muscle during the displacement procedure. Despite using a vertically driven arthrograph they did not offset the mass of the limb.

The difference in the results obtained from the horizontally driven arthrograph measurements was attributed to the stiffness measurements done relative to the equilibrium position. The authors claimed that the RA patients were rather less stiff objectively. Helliwell *et al.*, (1988) used a microprocessor-controlled arthrograph to measure the stiffness of the MCP joint in the abduction/adduction plane. These authors used a relatively smaller amplitude of displacement (8°) compared to previous work. The device they used was far more sophisticated compared to those used earlier, allowing an on-line analysis of hysteresis loops and manipulation of test conditions, so that the waveform shape, frequency and amplitude could be altered. In their results, they found that the patients with active RA showed stiffness values no greater than controls, which is surprising. The results did not indicate the status of the muscle, which might be a possible contributor to the negative result.

In another study, resistive torque was measured while applying a standard displacement to the finger over two seconds when maximum force of the fingers was measured using a Rigimeter (Rasker *et al.*, 1986). The study observed that the RA patients were stiffer, but the results were more widely scattered than for controls. The mean force values were found to be significantly lower in patients. The authors did not find any correlation between the force produced and stiffness.

Objective measurement of knee stiffness, until recently is done using Wartenburg modified pendulum test, which was commonly used to assess spasticity (Burks & Keegan, 2006; Valle *et al.*, 2006). Wartenburg's pendulum test was done with the participants sitting on a table with legs hanging freely. The examiner then raised their relaxed leg to horizontal position and then released the leg to swing freely. Irregularities in the motion of the swinging leg and a decrease in the number of oscillations indicated increased spasticity (Wartenburg, 1951).

A modified version of Wartenburg pendulum test was designed to minimize the amount of resistance from contracting muscles. The modified version was used to measure mechanical resistance of the knee and surrounding structures, indicating stiffness of the knee joint. Goniometers and motion analysis system were used along with the pendulum test for improved accuracy (Oatis *et al.*, 1995). This test was used in a few studies to measure knee joint stiffness objectively and the method offered objective measure of knee joint stiffness with high level of reliability (Oatis *et al.*, 1995; Burks & Keegan, 2006). However, the limitations of this method are – limited portability of the devices and it cannot be applied for joist other than the knee.

Passive knee stiffness was found to be significantly higher in RA patients, when studied using the pendulum test of Wartenberg. The knee was extended and let to swing passively, the trajectory of the leg providing kinematic measurements. This study also has found a moderate correlation between the severity of the disease and stiffness and has reported a decrease in the amplitude of the first flexion and first extension in RA patients. But no mention was made of any corrections for the mass of the limb. The result also suggests that there might be increase in the number of acto-myosin crossbridges at rest which get disrupted during the first cycle.

1.6. Contribution of Structures Other than the Joint

The imposed displacement to the joint not only offers information on the joint properties but also on the periarticular tissues, muscles and tendons, involved in the joint movement. Arthrographs have been used to quantify spasticity in hemiplegic subjects and the studies have shown marked increases in viscous and elastic stiffness in those patients (Joyce *et al.*, 1974). The relative contribution of various tissues to stiffness varies from joint to joint and also is dependent on the load applied to the joint at the time of the task (Johns & Wright, 1962). The loss of quadriceps muscle bulk following injury caused decreases in the non-elastic joint stiffness due to immobilization. The stiffness was found to return to normal levels after rehabilitation induced re-mobilization (Heerkens *et al.*, 1986, 1987). This study provides support to the theory that a significant change in any of the periarticular structure could change the passive resistance of the joint.

In RA patients, significant changes to the muscle bulk due to atrophy were reported (Steinberg & Wynn-Parry, 1961). There is evidence supporting the theory that RA causes pathological modifications of the muscles and connective tissues. Studies have shown that the grip strength is significantly reduced in RA patients (Helliwell *et al.*, 1987a, b; Alpiner *et al.*, 1995). RA induces changes in muscle fibre size, length, type and length ratio, angle and the physical properties of the muscle fibre and tendon attachment, even in the number of crossbridges (Alpiner *et al.*, 1995). The decrease in the contribution of muscle towards the total resistance to displacement could have offset any increased resistance contributed by the articular and periarticular structures, resulting in the disparity of the results compared to the earlier studies. If the total measured stiffness to a joint can be broken down experimentally and contribution of individual structure to the total stiffness studied, the individual contributors to arthritic stiffness could be determined.

1.7. Quantification of Stiffness

Few studies have been done to measure the physiological correlates of stiffness. In one study, the joint was driven through repeated sinusoidal movements at frequencies that were generally higher than could be achieved by voluntary effort (Joyce *et al.*, 1974). A repeating movement has the advantage that it is possible to measure force over a number of similar cycles, and separate the relevant force changes from other random fluctuations. Sinusoidal movements have the particular advantages that they are easy to generate, the methods of analysis are well understood and they bear some resemblance to spontaneous tremor. At rest, the passive components viz. elasticity and viscosity contribute to the total stiffness.

A system that contains viscosity, elasticity and inertia responds to sinusoidal movement with a force that is also a sinusoid and of constant phase with respect to the movement. At low frequencies the stiffness is mainly due to tissue elasticity. The resulting torque is in phase with position and is small (depending on the elastic constant). As the frequency increases, the resistive torque increases exponentially until it is 180° out of phase with position. At higher frequencies the stiffness therefore is due mainly to inertial forces (Burne *et al.*, 1995). At some intermediate frequency, the effects of the inertia and the elasticity are equal but 180° out of phase, so the forces can cancel each other; the system is then said to be at resonance. When the system is unrestrained, it oscillates with a natural frequency that is the same as this resonant frequency. The residual resistance is due to the viscous or frictional component (Joyce *et al.*, 1974).

1.8. Reflex Contribution to Joint Stiffness

It has been hypothesized that the stretch reflex has a role in the determination of viscoelastic properties of muscle and therefore of the limb. Resultant limb characteristics are the superposition of the contributions of the limb's passive elements, muscle contraction level and active reflexes. Since information on force, length and its derivatives converges on the α-MN, it is possible that the reflex has a role in the regulation of the combination of force and length - viz. stiffness. Houk, *et al.*, (1981) have shown that stiffness can be regulated by a simple summation of excitatory and inhibitory signals at the level of the α-MN. What has been debated is the degree to which these characteristics can be controlled by manipulation of the reflex. They suggested that neither muscle length nor force is regulated as individual variables but that muscle stiffness is maintained relatively constant by skeletomotor reflexes.

Many studies have been done over the years to explain stretch reflex mechanisms, yet its origin, characteristics and role are still much debated (Hunter & Kearney, 1982; Toft *et al.*, 1989; Stein & Kearney, 1995). The stretch reflex is a necessary response of the system which is absolutely vital for the execution and regulation of locomotion and voluntary movements (Crago *et al.*, 1976; Nakazawa *et al.*, 1997; Cathers *et al.*, 2004).

1.9. Anatomy of the Stretch Reflex

Skeletal muscle has two major group I receptors, namely muscle spindles and Golgi tendon organs (GTO) which are involved in the transmission of the stretch signal and muscle tension to the spinal cord. Muscle spindles are a mixture of sensory neurons and muscle fibres (intrafusal fibres), which are the only contractile sense organ of the body (Marsden *et al.*, 1976). Muscle spindles sense the changes in muscle length and the GTO senses the force changes in the muscle due to contraction (Hasan & Stuart, 1984; Al-Falahe *et al.*, 1990). Primary Ia afferents of the muscle spindles detect changes in length and velocity, while the secondary group II afferents are sensitive primarily to the length change. When muscle forces change, the GTO in the junction of muscle fibres and muscle tendon detect the change and relay the information to the spinal cord through Ib afferent fibres.

When a muscle is lengthened or stretched, the spindles are stretched, which is sensed by Ia and group II afferents and relayed to the spinal cord. The changes in the muscle length and rate of change are the information sent to the spinal cord α-MNs innervating the muscle then fire, resulting in a graded muscle contraction and increased force of contraction. Thus by increasing the force output of the muscle, the stretch reflex resists the muscle stretch.

When a muscle is shortened, the central regions of the muscle spindle refrain from contracting, thus letting the spindles remain slack. When α-MNs fire to contract the muscle, the γ-MNs (fusimotor system) also fire simultaneously to contract the polar regions of the spindle. This results in the stretching of the middle sensory region (alpha-gamma co-activation). Thus by always maintaining the spindle length parallel to the muscle length, the sensitivity of the spindle remains unaltered (Gordon & Ghez, 1991).

1.10. Reflex Studies Employing a Phasic Stretch Stimulus

Stretch reflex studies are commonly based on phasic signals, which are sudden brief stretch perturbations to the muscle. Phasic signals include ramp stretches (Gottlieb & Agarwal, 1979; Berardelli *et al.*, 1982; Thilmann *et al.*, 1991; Kirsch *et al.*, 1993), pulses (Marsden *et al.*, 1978; Noth *et al.*, 1991), tendon vibration (Cody *et al.*, 1987) and a step-wise increase of the torque signal. Phasic perturbations are typically high frequency signals and elicit a short burst of stretch response called the phasic stretch reflex (PSR). The PSR elicits an early, short latency response (M1) and a longer latency response (M2) (Marsden *et al.*, 1974, 1976; Bawa & McKenzie, 1981; Matthews, 1989; Thilmann *et al.*, 1991).

The two reflexes are thought to be mediated by two different pathways, a short latency pathway involving the spinal cord (Marsden *et al.*, 1978) and the long latency pathway involving transcortical pathways (Neilson & Neilson, 1978; Matthews, 1993). The PSR is generally quantified in terms of the reflex gain and latency. The advantage of using a phasic stimulus in reflex studies is the brief duration of the stretch which aids in the clear distinction of M1 and M2 responses in time. The responses to the stimulus are then quantified (Gottlieb & Agarwal, 1979) in terms of reflex gain and latency.

Lee, *et al.*,(1978) used a phasic stimulus in wrist muscles and reported reflex delays of 30 and 58 ms respectively, for short and long loop pathways. In the ankle joint, the reflex delays have been reported in the range of 35-45 and 60-80 ms respectively for M1 and M2 responses (Kearney & Hunter, 1982). The difference in the latencies in the upper limb and lower limb is considered mainly due to the distance of the muscle from the spinal cord, which reflects the conduction time of the reflex transmission (Latash, 1993). There are also a few studies that suggest that the latencies could be influenced by parameters such as acceleration of the stretch (Bozec *et al.*, 1987), height of the subject (Stam & van Creval, 1989) and level of muscle activation (Toft *et al.*, 1989).

Though it remained a popular stimulus for stretch studies, the PSR failed to produce consistent results across studies. The reflex delay and amplitude of the responses varied significantly between experiments even while using the same joint (Gottlieb & Agarwal,

1979; Kearney & Hunter, 1982; Fellows *et al.*, 1993). The disadvantage of using the PSR is the difficulty in controlling the frequency content of the stretch response. A further problem with phasic stimuli is their high frequency content which may be beyond the stretch reflex system's linear encoding range. This could possibly result in misleading results (Neilson, 1993). None of the studies using the PSR attempted to standardize the frequency content of the stretch stimulus delivered by different methods, which makes comparison between studies difficult. The studies using the PSR have left a lot for speculation including characterization of the subcomponents of the reflex system (Matthews, 1993). To date, the PSR has failed to explain the functional role of the stretch reflex.

1.11. Reflex Studies Employing Tonic Stretch Stimulus

Unlike the PSR perturbation, continuous perturbation with low frequency sinusoidal signals produces a tonic stretch reflex (TSR). The reflex response to a continuous stretch is called TSR (Neilson, 1973). Stein (1995) suggested that the TSR is the combined response from spinal and supraspinal activity. While PSR results in muscle twitch, TSR results in sustained muscle contraction (Latash, 1993). Neilson (1993) has shown that the TSR response can be differentiated in resting and contracting muscle.

The TSR, produced in response to slow stretch is a long latency muscle contraction. It can be characterized using reflex threshold and gain. Cross-correlational analysis is used to separate the linear reflex component from the non-linear background component of the EMG signal. The phase difference between the torque and the position is used as an indicator of reflex latency in this analysis (Gordon & Ghez, 1991).

An advantage of using sinusoidal perturbations in reflex studies is that these signals have a well-characterized frequency content, which makes it possible to relate the TSR response and reflex delays with the frequency content of the perturbation signal. Dynamic responses of the reflex pathway can be easily explored by changing the frequency content of the stimulus, thus enabling studies on transmission characteristics of the reflex pathways over a range of stimulus frequencies.

Sinusoidal perturbations are commonly employed in TSR studies (Matthews & Stein, 1969; Burke *et al.*, 1971; Joyce *et al.*, 1974; Rack *et al.*, 1983). It has been demonstrated that if a system generates multiple peaks at different latencies for a rapid stretch, it is also capable of generating a sinusoidal response to sinusoidal stretches (Neilson & Neilson, 1978). Sinusoidal signals are easy to generate and they involve no sudden movements so the stretch will be more physiological (Rack *et al.*, 1978).

A disadvantage of using sinusoidal perturbations is that the regularity of the signal may result in nonlinearity in the reflex response (Agarwal & Gottlieb, 1977). However, the frequency range that can be linearly encoded and transmitted by the nervous system may only be up to about 10 Hz (Cathers *et al.*, 1999). The reflex responses above this frequency range may be distorted by the transmission process and might be nonlinear (Stein *et al.*, 1972; Cathers *et al.*, 1999). The predictability of the signal may allow the subject to modulate the voluntary action (Hunter & Kearney, 1982). However, studies have shown that it is impossible to produce coherent voluntary movements above 2 Hz (Neilson, 1972). While it also has been suggested that such problems can be overcome by giving careful instructions to the subjects (Cathers *et al.*, 1999), another study suggests that it is possible to track sinusoidal signals up to 7 Hz (Cathers *et al.*, 1996).

Alternatively, stochastic input or random perturbations are also used in some studies to elicit the TSR (Agarwal & Gottlieb, 1977; Gottlieb & Agarwal, 1979; Hunter & Kearney, 1982; Kearney & Hunter, 1982). The randomness of this signal helps avoiding these predictive or preprogrammed responses and thus serves as a better alternative for sinusoidal perturbations (Hunter & Kearney, 1982). However, a recent study found that there is a consistent difference present in TSR responses evoked by sinusoidal and random perturbations and sinusoidal stretches yield a higher gain and greater phase advance in the response (Cathers *et al.*, 1999).

Kearney *et al.*, (1997) applied a pseudorandom binary sequence of angular perturbations to the ankle and used a nonlinear parallel-cascade system identification technique to separate overall stiffness into intrinsic and reflexive components. Hunter *et al.*, (1982) described the intrinsic stiffness as a linear second order system. High frequency, vibratory inputs have been shown to inhibit stretch reflexes (Matthews, 1984). Therefore, the perturbation signals need to be selected carefully to effectively determine the reflex stiffness.

Both short and long latency pathways could influence the TSR, as for the PSR. Since the stretch is continuous in the TSR, the reflex magnitude and reflex delay produce a single net response that is a combination of both short and long loop pathways (Neilson & Neilson, 1978). The latencies of the response vary with the joint under study, owing to the varying distances from the spinal cord. Matthews (1993) has used sinusoidal perturbations on biceps and finger muscles and reported the latencies to be 32 and 62 ms respectively.

While the PSR may be quantified by EMG amplitude and reflex latency, the TSR may be quantified by reflex coherence square, gain and phase with respect to the stretch perturbation. Reflex coherence square is a measure of the proportion of the variance between the stretch input and the linearly correlated output response. Reflex gain is a ratio of amplitude of output signal (linearly correlated component of the rectified EMG) to the input signal (stretch) and reflex phase is a measure of time delay between the stretch and reflex response, expressed in degrees. Measuring the TSR in a contracting muscle is complex, as the reflex responses are contaminated with background muscle activity (Neilson & Neilson, 1978).

1.12. Joint Dynamics

The stretch reflex partly determines the viscoelastic properties of muscle and joint. Therefore, joint function and limb movement are the superposition of passive elements, muscle contraction level and active reflexes. The reflex is hypothesized to regulate muscle force and length and therefore joint stiffness. This might be due to the fact that the derivatives of the muscle length and force converge on the α-MN. Houk, *et al.*, (1981) have shown that stiffness can be regulated by a simple summation of excitatory and inhibitory signals at the level of the α-MN.

A recent study by the authors explored the reflex mediated changes and mechanical changes in RA affected joint employing TSR, induced by sinusoidal perturbations. The results suggest a disproportionate loss of the large diameter afferent response and significant loss of neural drive to the motor unit population. The increased stiffness observed in contracting muscle and not in the resting muscle prompts the suggestion that the increased joint stiffness in RA is due to changes in the mechanical properties of the active muscle-joint system rather than changes in the reflex properties (Rajagopalan & Burne, 2010). However, further studies are needed to tease out the mechanism involved.

1.13. Task Dependent Modulation of Stretch Reflexes

Spinal reflexes, for a long time were viewed as simple, stereotypic motor patterns, whose magnitude can be related to the strength of the initiating stimulus with limited scope for modification. This view was in contradiction to the greater adaptive possibilities shown by the behavior of longer latency reflexes and voluntary reactions. This prompted a barrage of studies on the modulation of short and long latency reflexes (Forsberg, 1979; Akazawa *et al.*, 1983; Capaday & Stein, 1986, 1987; Edamura *et al.*, 1991; Duysens *et al.*, 1992; Brooke *et al.*, 1995). In normal subjects the joint stiffness acts to maintain constant stiffness. This can be deduced using resonant frequency (Sinkjaer & Hayashi, 1989). The H-reflex was found to be profoundly attenuated during passive (Mcilroy *et al.*, 1992) and active (Brooke *et al.*, 1992) leg movements, compared with the reflexes evoked from a stationary limb. These studies proved that spinal reflexes could be subjected to a high degree of modulation during simple motor tasks and that the pattern of modulation can be specifically altered for different functional requirements of the motor task (Stein & Capaday, 1988).

The central nervous system is hypothesized to regulate the sensitivity of the stretch reflex according to the changes in the muscular force. The magnitude of the stretch reflex was found to increase with increasing motor unit activity and vice versa (Kimura *et al.*, 2003). The possible mechanism has been ascribed to the pre-synaptic inhibition of Ia afferent activity and/or the modulation of muscle spindle sensitivity (Gollhofer *et al.*, 1998).

Studies on upper limb reflex activity have explored central-peripheral interactions regulating arm or finger movements (Caccia *et al.*, 1973; Evans *et al.*, 1989; Matthews, 1989; Edamura *et al.*, 1991; Chen & Ashby, 1993; Nakazawa *et al.*, 1997; Zehr & Stein, 1999; Zehr & Chua, 2000; Zehr *et al.*, 2001; Xia *et al.*, 2005). However, most of the studies done in upper limbs were on reflexes mediated by fast cutaneous afferents. Little attention has been given to the task- and phase-dependent modulation of the muscle afferents during rhythmic, fine motor tasks (Dufresne *et al.*, 1980; Johnson *et al.*, 1991; Kimura *et al.*, 2003; Xia *et al.*, 2005). Many investigators (Stein & Kearney, 1995; Brooke *et al.*, 1997; McCrea, 2001) have reported modulation of spinal stretch reflex responses in the lower limbs during locomotion. In these muscles also it was found that increased reflex gain follows greater muscle activation, thereby increasing the joint stiffness (Akazawa *et al.*, 1983; Doemges & Rack, 1992).

Previous experiments have used brief stretches and have studied the contribution of the tissues to joint dynamics. The muscles and other elastic periarticular structures influence passive joint mechanics (Proske *et al.*, 1993). They offer an elastic resistance to displacement (Agarwal & Gottlieb, 1977; Lin & Sabbahi, 1998) and contribute to the overall joint resistance to imposed movement (Rack, 1981). These periarticular structures provide a strong viscoelastic resistance, increasing the overall stiffness. These structures are also sensitive to the frequency with which the joint is displaced (Purslow, 1989; Carter *et al.*, 1993; Kirsch *et al.*, 1994b; Mirbagheri *et al.*, 2000).

Even though studies support task dependent modulation during rhythmic limb movement, the neural mechanism and the patterns of reflex modulation are yet to be revealed clearly. Documenting the pattern of stretch reflex control during normal limb movement could help explain the neural control mechanisms on which the volitional behaviors are based (Brooke *et al.*, 1997). The degree of reflex modulation has been found to change with the motor task and the phase of the task.

Several autogenic neural pathways are said to mediate stretch reflexes. The autogenic muscle receptors are the primary and secondary endings in muscle spindles sensitive to stretch and the GTO, sensitive to tension. The entire control system termed 'motor servo', continuously conveys graded amounts of inhibitory and excitatory regulation to large α-MNs. Smaller γ-MNs regulate spindle-receptor discharge in the muscle spindles (Houk, 1979).

Even though extensive studies on the neurophysiological mechanisms underlying stretch reflexes have provided many valuable insights, the functional importance of the stretch reflex in the neuromuscular system remains a matter of controversy. It was thought that the function of stretch and unloading reflexes was to regulate the muscle length against changes in the mechanical load, thereby providing load compensation (Merton, 1953), until an alternative concept started evolving with the work of Nichols, *et al.*, (1976). In this study, they provided evidence to support the notion that it is the ratio of force change to length change (ie. stiffness) that was being regulated not the individual variables. The stretch reflex, during changing background contraction, has been hypothesized to compensate for the nonlinearities in mechanical properties thereby regulating muscle stiffness. There is evidence supporting the theory that the EMG responses are mainly regulated by the motor system rather than the differences in the reflex tuning (Dyhre-Poulson *et al.*, 1991).

Mirbagheri *et al.*, (2000) found that intrinsic stiffness increased with contraction level, but reflex stiffness was maximal at low contraction levels and then decreased. They also observed various joint angle related differences between intrinsic and reflexive stiffness. Reflex stiffness gain was found to decrease as the mean velocity of the perturbation increased, and intrinsic stiffness was invariant to this change in velocity. As the frequency increases beyond 10 Hz, the reflex activation (EMG) will continue to increase, but the force of the muscle will not increase because of the low-pass filter nature of muscle mechanics.

1.14. Contribution of Intrinsic Muscle Properties to Joint Stiffness

Physical assessment, grip test, and subjective pain rating using an analog scale (Arnett *et al.*, 1988b; Alpiner *et al.*, 1995) are currently used to monitor the severity and progression of RA. However, these are based on the subjective perceptions. The clinical course of the disease can only be monitored by objectively measuring the most sensible outcomes of the progressive worsening of the motor function.

The stretch-evoked force response of a muscle could be due to intrinsic stiffness of the contracting muscle, generating force via sliding filaments and acto-myosin crossbridges supplemented by the reflex responses. The motor system achieves precision control by compensating for the changes in the internal and external loads that interfere with intended movements. Passive muscular resistance, co-contractions and even inertia may contribute to the total load (Akazawa *et al.*, 1983).

Load compensation depends mainly on the precise detection of changes in muscle length and tension. Such mechanisms rely on the proprioceptive information relayed by the peripheral receptors, such as muscle spindles and Golgi tendon organs. The motor commands to the force-generating skeletal muscles are modified by the central nervous system in accordance with the afferent feedback on the changes in muscle length and tension (Riemann & Lephart, 2002).

The common property attributed to skeletal muscles was viscoelasticity. The elastic property of the muscle provides the length-dependent tension response whereas the velocity-dependent tension response is provided by the viscous property. The viscoelastic structures provide the muscles with different types of characteristic tension responses during and after the changes in the muscle lengths (Buchthal *et al.*, 1951).

1.15. Thixotropy and Joint Stiffness

During a passive stretch-release cycle, the muscle tension is higher during lengthening than during shortening. When a muscle is stretched sinusoidally it will resist the stretch with its viscous and elastic forces. The viscous stiffness would be at the same frequency as the stretch, but with increasing frequencies the phase of the stiffness will lag behind the stretch (Axelson & Hagbarth, 2001). This phenomenon gives rise to hysteresis.

Experimentally, a hysteresis loop can be obtained by plotting the joint angle against resistive tension produced by the joint, for a given stretch stimulus (Figure 2). A pure elastic system has no hysteresis and so the hysteresis plot will return a straight line. However, deviation from this straight line during flexion and extension implies the loss of energy between the shortening and lengthening periods of the muscle. The amount of energy lost is indicated by the area of the loop. Factors such as rate of crossbridge formation can influence the hysteresis area due to changes in the viscous resistance and thus loss of energy. A reduced rate of crossbridge cycling results in an increased viscous stiffness and more energy is used up to detach the bonds. This increase in viscous stiffness is represented by increased hysteresis area. Crossbridge formation depends on the past history of the muscle length change, so the hysteresis area can provide a measure of changes in muscle thixotropy over time.

When the skeletal muscles are maintained at a lengthened position, following a stretch, the resisting muscle tension slowly declines to reach a steady state level, which is termed *stress relaxation*. On the contrary, if the muscle is contracted and maintained at short length, the resistive tension gradually increases: *stress recovery* (Axelson, 1999; Axelson & Hagbarth, 2001, 2003; Axelson, 2004, 2005a). Viscoelastic properties of the muscle produces history-dependent after-effects and the crossbridge mechanisms seem to be the predominant reason for this effect (Butler *et al.*, 1978). However, some authors have suggested structures other than muscles, like skin (Finlay, 1978) and unfolding of titin, a muscle protein, also could contribute to the effect. Of particular interest are those domains of the titin protein that unfold during stretch and recoil during shortening (Minajeva *et al.*, 2001). Titin has been hypothesized to be the major contributor to the elastic behaviour of the skeletal muscles (Linke, 2000).

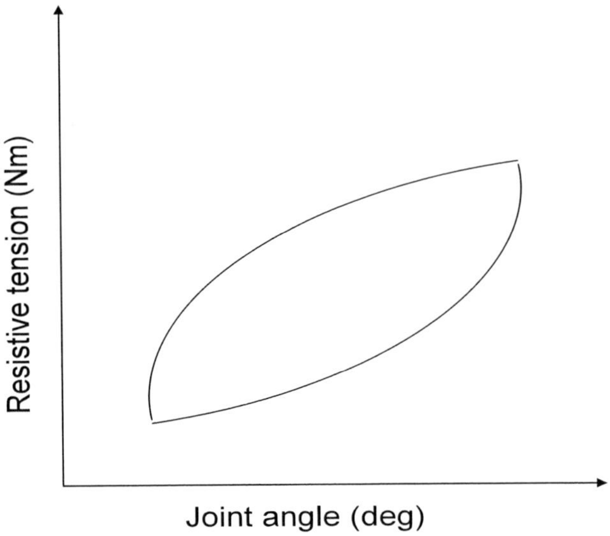

Figure 1.2. Theoretical representation of a hysteresis loop

Hill (1968) proposed that there is a short-range stiffness to the skeletal muscle at rest generated by stable cross bridging of actin with myosin, which he proposed are broken during stretch and reform again when the muscle is relaxed. In their study on the amphibian skeletal muscle, Buchthal *et al.*,(1951) found the stiffness to decrease during stretching movement and to return after a short rest. As a response to imposed movements to the ankle, Hufschimidt *et al.*, (1987) found an initial sharp increase in the joint torque which they implied to be due to short-term stiffness. They found passive movement or voluntary contraction or even electrical stimulation can reduce the short-term stiffness temporarily.

The thixotropic properties of the muscle may be modified by the recent history of movement (Hagbarth *et al.*, 1985) and therefore have significance for voluntary movements (Axelson & Hagbarth, 2001; Axelson, 2005b). The system may change its physical properties when shaken mechanically (Lakie *et al.*, 1984; Proske *et al.*, 1993). Since the thixotropy of the muscle is primarily due to the dynamic process of crossbridge formation, both amplitude and frequency of a perturbation can influence the state of the bonds and thus stiffness.

Clinical evidence suggests subjective stiffness in RA patients is affected by their previous history of muscle activity. Patients report benefit from limbering-up exercises after a long period of inactivity (Klepper, 2003; Stenstrom & Minor, 2003). Warming-up procedures such as stretching of limbs are reported to reduce joint stiffness and increase joint range of motion (Harvey *et al.*, 2002; LaRoche & Connolly, 2006).

Following active or passive movement, resting human muscle shows a significant and progressive increase in stiffness over the time it remains in the passive state (Lakie & Robson, 1988b). Lakie et al., (1984) proposed that increased stiffness observed in certain pathological disorders could be due to the 'exaggerated' thixotropic properties of the muscle. Thixotropy has been studied in pathological conditions such as spasticity following stroke (Vattanasilp *et al.*, 2000), hemiplegia (Brown *et al.*, 1987) and tetraplegia (Walsh, 1992b). In RA, it is possible that the thixotropic property is augmented and could contribute to joint stiffness. It remains to be elucidated whether the inactivity influenced by joint pain or pathological changes due to RA results in increased thixotropy.

1.16. Modification of Sensory Perception at the Joint

Active periods of RA are characterized by stiffness especially in the morning time, loss of range of motion of the joints with or without pain. Many studies evaluating arthritic patients emphasized that the stiffness measurement was done on a purely subjective basis (Kellgren & Lawrence, 1957; Lansbury, 1958). But some studies have found no demonstrable objective stiffness that matches the subjective claim (Unsworth *et al.*, 1982; Helliwell *et al.*, 1988). This discrepancy between subjective impression and objective measurement could be due to miscommunication between the patient and the assessor. The patient's interpretation of stiffness could be different from that of the professional interpretation.

Since the sensory signals are synthesized by the peripheral anatomical structures that are in varying states of dysfunction as the result of inflammation there is a possibility of misrepresentation of the perceived stiffness. There have been suggestions that patients confuse stiffness with limitation of movement or stiffness might be an outcome of muscle weakness (Wright & Johns, 1960a). It may also be that the original sensation of stiffness is not perceived properly due to aberrant sensory information sent from the periphery (Helliwell *et al.*, 1987b). The painful stimuli from the joints might modify the sensitivity of mechanoreceptors in joint, ligaments, and capsules at the spinal level (Harvey, 1987). It has been reported that a pure analgesic is capable of relieving morning stiffness in RA, which could be taken as a support for Harvey's hypothesis (Emery & Gibson, 1986). All these suggest a need for objective measures of stiffness and pain perception.

The main complaint of a patient suffering from RA, besides stiffness, is pain. The pain results from the inflammatory process. According to literature, continuous pain input from the periphery causes central sensitization, resulting in hyperalgesia (Coggeshall *et al.*, 1983; Andersen *et al.*, 2005b). The afferent pain input could be the source of the reflex activity which could cause reflex stiffness of the affected joint.

1.17. Peripheral Nociceptive Mechanisms in RA

The study of the receptors of peripheral nociceptive inputs could shed light on some of the intricate interplay of sensory afferents mediating signal transduction. The mechanism that causes the peripheral inputs to be amplified as central sensitization, could well be the reason for excessive reflex activity in the vicinity of the inflamed joint (Koltzenburg *et al.*, 1994; Andrew & Greenspan, 1999; Staud *et al.*, 2001; Winkelstein, 2004).

Nociception has been defined (Loeser, 2000) as 'the detection of tissue damage by specialised transducers connected to Aδ- and C- fibres. Anatomically this process occurs predominantly peripherally and involves the nociceptor neurons, which terminate in the dorsal horn of the spinal cord'.

Unlike most other receptors, nociceptors become increasingly sensitive with continuing or repeated stimulation. When tissues become injured or inflamed, as with a sunburn or infection, they release chemicals called prostaglandins and leukotrienes that make nociceptors much more sensitive. Sensitized nociceptors react to even gentle stimuli, such as a breeze or a caress, causing pain (Sandkuhler & Liu, 1998).

1.18. Pain and Reflexes

Hugon (1973) correlated withdrawal reflexes with psycho-physiological studies of pain. He studied the relationship between pain perception and the effect of tactile and nociceptive input on nociceptive reflex responses. Willer (1977) was able to relate the pain perception to reflex thresholds. Subsequent studies resulted in the idea of using withdrawal reflexes as an 'objective' physiological correlate of experimental pain (Willer, 1984; DeBroucker & al, 1989; Andersen *et al.*, 2000; Bouhassira *et al.*, 2003; Andersen *et al.*, 2005a). According to these studies, the pain perceived by the subject was found to be directly proportional to the size of the withdrawal reflex.

Helliwell (1994) speculated that in RA, continuous activation of C- fibre afferents may alter at a spinal level the sensory threshold for articular mechano-receptors. The speculation was based on animal studies which showed that chronic pain stimuli transmitted by unmyelinated C-fibres may alter the receptor characteristics for mechanical stimuli transmitted by myelinated Aδ- fibres. The peripheral tissue inflammation produces long-term changes in the synaptic efficacy in the dorsal horn involving cellular mechanisms. This could to be an adaptive response prompting induction of tissue repair mechanisms.

1.19. Summary

The stiffness in RA affected joints could be purely due to peripheral changes. However, since there is the involvement of continuous peripheral nociceptive inputs (Andrew & Greenspan, 1999) and central sensitization due to expansion of reflex receptors (Coggeshall *et al.*, 1983), there is a possibility that reflexes could contribute to the effective stiffness. Joint dynamics can be investigated by studying the relationship between the joint torque and joint angle. Cross-correlational analysis using gain and phase as a function of frequency is considered a good experimental approach (Kearney & Hunter, 1982; Sinkjaer & Hayashi, 1989; Sinkjaer & Magnussen, 1994; Kirsch & Kearney, 1997). Gain quantifies the reflex magnitude and phase, the reflex delay.

The pathological modification of muscle viscosity and tissue elasticity were considered as the physiological correlate of OJS. The studies so far provided diametrically opposite results on the objective stiffness measures in RA patients. While some authors found the RA joints stiffer than the controls (Wright & Johns, 1960a, 1961; Backlund & Tiselius, 1967), few studies reported lack of objective stiffness in RA (Helliwell *et al.*, 1988; Helliwell, 1994; Helliwell, 1997). Haigh, *et al.*,(2003) state that measurement of OJS does not relate to that experienced by RA patients. The contentious issue of OJS needs to be approached using methods that would bring out the physiological correlates of the contributors to the stiffness.

Substantial contribution to chronic pain in RA arises from the component of pain which is due to local inflammation. Consequent to arthritis the nociceptive system undergoes changes at peripheral and central nervous levels (Schaible *et al.*, 1991). It has been proposed that the common clinical complaint of subjective rigidity and immobility be described as PJS since it has been shown that measures of OJS do not relate to subjective experience (Wendler *et al.*, 2001; Haigh *et al.*, 2003). The CNS is capable of generating a feedback-dependent state which can result in pathological sensations such as pain and stiffness that are to some extent independent of the initial peripheral pathology.

Quite a few studies have suggested a neural reorganisation due to continuous activation of C-fibre afferents. Helliwell, *et al.*,(1998) have shown that objectively quantified articular stiffness is not related to subjective stiffness using arthrography measurements. Coggeshall et al., have suggested when there is expansion of reflex receptive fields, there are not only changes to the resting muscle electrical activity but also to normally innocuous joint movements. They have found that more motor units are recruited due to the articular activity following experimentally induced acute joint inflammation (Coggeshall *et al.*, 1983).

Impaired muscle function and reduced functionality are frequently observed in patients suffering from RA. Yet, they have not been quantified effectively. It is not clear whether the reduced muscle endurance has a physiological basis or it is just the involuntary, subjective reaction to pain and/or inflammation. Pathological changes following RA results in problems relating to muscle strength, endurance and balance/coordination (Ekdahl *et al.*, 1989). Muscle involvement in the pathology of RA has been studied using biopsy, dynamometry, ultrastructural scans and electromyography (Ekdahl *et al.*, 1989; Ekdahl, 1990; Ekdahl & Broman, 1992a; Lamontagne *et al.*, 1998; de Palma *et al.*, 2000; Agrawal *et al.*, 2003; Lindehammar & Lindvall, 2004; Escalante *et al.*, 2005), but the physiological aspects need elucidation.

The acto-myosin bonds or the degree of muscle contraction at a given moment largely regulates the intrinsic muscle stiffness. It is likely that preceding reflex-mediated stiffness also could have a role in the regulation (Johansson *et al.*, 1993). If joint afferents have a significant role in the regulation of reflex-mediated muscle stiffness, they also may have significance for intrinsic muscle stiffness. Therefore, the changes in the crossbridge mediated muscle properties can also be influenced by the preceding status of reflex activity. Investigation of these properties in RA affected joint may provide insight on the mechanism that regulates the overall stiffness.

Animal studies have proved that nociceptor activation can lead to increased fusimotor firing (Kniffki *et al.*, 1978; Appelberg *et al.*, 1983). Significant increases in the mechanical stretch reflex (ankle torque) and EMG responses have been reported from soleus and tibialis anterior muscles in humans following noxious electrical stimulation (Matre *et al.*, 1998). A detailed study of the CMR might provide a clear insight on the contribution of nociceptive transmission to the pathology of RA. Chronic pain and inflammatory metabolites in RA may alter the threshold for the articular mechanoreceptor thus permitting the transmission of misleading information, which might be perceived as stiffness by the patient.

There are substantial gains to be made in arthritis research generally if objective diagnostic criteria and measurement techniques are developed. Such techniques open the way to providing objective methods for acute assessment of new drugs and other forms of therapy. Further, neuro-biomechanical techniques can clarify the underlying mechanisms contributing to disability thus providing potentially new criteria for diagnosis, monitoring of disease progression and identification of disease subtypes. Significant flow on benefits for other research arises from this type of advance. Objective measures of the clinical condition should be of great benefit in establishing links between arthritis and its underlying genetic and biological mechanisms, currently areas of intense research effort internationally.

References

ACR. (2002). Guidelines for the management of rheumatoid arthritis: update. In *Arthritis Rheum*, pp. 328-346. American college of rheumatology subcommittee.

Agarwal, G. C. & Gottlieb, G. L. (1977). Compliance of the human ankle joint. *Transactions on ASME Journal Biomedical Engineering, 99*, 166-170.

Agrawal, V., Husain, N., Das, S. K. & Bagchi, M. (2003). Muscle involvement in rheumatoid arthritis: Clinical and histological characteristics and review of literature. *Journal of Indian Rheumatological association, 11*, 98-103.

Akazawa, K., Milner, T. E. & Stein, R. B. (1983). Modulation of reflex EMG and stiffness in response to stretch of human finger muscle. *Journal of Neurophysiology, 49*, 16-27.

Al-Falahe, N. A., Nagoaka, M. & Vallbo, A. B. (1990). Response profiles of human muscle afferents during active finger movements. *Brain, 113*, 325-346.

Alpiner, N., Oh, T. H., Hinderer, S. R. & Brander, V. A. (1995). Rehabiliation in joint and connective tissue disease. I. Systemic diseases. *Archives of Physiology and Medical Rehabilitation, 76*, S32-S40.

Amick, L. D. (2005). Muscle atrophy in rheumatoid arthritis: An electrodiagnostic study. *Arthritis and Rheumatism, 3*, 54 - 63.

Amir, R. & Devor, M. (2000). Functional cross-excitation between afferent A- and C-neurons in dorsal root ganglia. *Neuroscience, 95*, 189-195.

Andersen, O. K., Finnerup, N. B., Spaich, E. G., Jensen, T. S. & Nielson, L. A. (2004). Expansion of nociceptive withdrawal reflex receptive fields in spinal cord injured humans. *Clinical Neurophysiology, 115*, 2798-2810.

Andersen, O. K., Jensen, L. M., Brennum, J. & Arendt-Nielson, L. (1994). Evidence for central summation of C and Aδ nociceptive activity in man. *Pain, 59*, 273-280.

Andersen, O. K., Nielson, T. G., Matre, D., Nielson, L. A. & Schomburg, E. D. (2000). Interaction between cutaneous and muscle afferent activity in polysynaptic reflex pathway: A human experimental study. *Pain, 84*, 29-36.

Andersen, O. K., Sonnenborg, F. A. & Nielson, L. A. (2001). Reflex receptive fields for human withdrawal refelxes elicited by non-painful electrical stimulation of the foot sole. *Clinical Neurophysiology, 112*, 641-649.

Andersen, O. K., Spaich, E. G., Madeleine, P. & Nielson, L. A. (2005a). Gradual enlargement of human withdrawal reflex receptive fields following repetitive painful stimulation. *Brain Res, 1042*, 194-204.

Andersen, O. K., Spaich, E. G., Madeleine, P. & Nielson, L. A. (2005b). Gradual enlargement of human withdrawal reflex receptive fields following repetive painful stimulation. *Brain Research, 1042*, 194-204.

Andrew, D. & Greenspan, J. D. (1999). Mechanical and heat sensitization of cutaneous nociceptors after peripheral inflammation in the rat. *Journal of Neurophysiology, 82*, 2649-2656.

Appelberg, B., Hulliger, M., Johansson, H. & Sojka, P. (1983). Actions on γ- motoneurones elicited by electrical stimulation of group I muscle afferent fibres in the hind limb of the cat. *Journal of Physiology, 335*, 237-253.

Arendt-Nielson, L., Andersen, O. K. & Jensen, T. S. (1996). Brief., prolonged and repeated stimuli applied to hyperalgesic skin areas: a psychophysical study. *Brain Research, 712*, 165-167.

Arnett, F. C., Edworthy, S. M., Bloch, D. A., McShane, D. J., Fries, J. F., Cooper, N. S., Healy, L. A. & Kaplan, S. R. (1988a). The American rheumatism association 1987 revised criteria for the classification of rheumatoid arthritis. *Arthritis and Rheumatism, 31*, 315-324.

Arnett, F. C., Edworthy, S. M., Bloch, D. A., McShane, D. J., Fries, J. F., Cooper, N. S., Healy, L. A. & Kaplan, S. R. (1988b). The American rheumatism association 1987 revised criteria for the classification of rheumatoid arthritis. *Arthritis Rheum, 31*, 315-324.

Arokoski, M. H., Arokoski, J. P. A., Haara, M., Kankaanpaa, M., Vesterienen, M., Niemitukia, L. H. & Helminen, H. J. (2002). Hip muscle strength and muscle cross sectional area in men with and without hip arhtritis. *J Rheumatol, 29*, 2185-2195.

Axelson, H. W. (1999). Signs of muscle thixotropy during human ballistic wrist joint movements. *Journal of Applied Physiology*.

Axelson, H. W. (2004). Human motor compensations for thixotropy-dependent changes in muscular resting after moderate joint movements. *Acta Physiol Scand, 182*, 295-304.

Axelson, H. W. (2005a). Signs of muscle muscle thixotropy during human ballistic wrist joint movements. *Journal of Applied Physiology, 99*, 1922-1929.

Axelson, H. W. (2005b). Signs of muscle thixotropy during human ballistic wrist joint movements. *J Appl Physiol, 99*, 1922-1929.

Axelson, H. W. & Hagbarth, K. E. (2001). Human motor control consequences of thixotropic changes in muscular short-range stiffness. *J Physiol, 535*, 279-288.

Axelson, H. W. & Hagbarth, K. E. (2003). Human motor compensations for thixotropy-dependent changes in resting wrist joint position after large joint movements. *Acta Physiol Scand, 179*, 389-398.

Backlund, L. & Tiselius, P. (1967). Objective measurement of joint stiffness in rheumatoid arthritis. *Acta Rheumatologica Scandinavica, 13*, 275-288.

Bawa, P. & McKenzie, D. C. (1981). Contribution of joint and cutaneous afferents to long-latency reflexes in man. *Brain Research, 211*, 185-189.

Becker, J. C. & Thakor, N. V. (1988). A study of the range of motion of human fingers with application to anthropomorphic designs. *IEEE Trans Biomed Eng 35*, 110-117.

Bekkelund, S. I., Torbergsen, T., Husby, G. & Mellgren, S. I. (1999). Myopathy and neuropathy in rheumatoid arthritis. A quantitative controlled electromyographic study. *J Rheumatol, 26*, 2348-2351.

Berardelli, A., Hallet, M., Kaufman, M. P., Fine, E., Berenberg, W. & Simon, S. R. (1982). Stretch reflexes of triceps surae in normal man. *Journal of Neurology, Neurosurgery and Psychiatry, 45*, 513-525.

Berg, H. E., Larsson, L. & Tesch, P. A. (1997). Lower limb skeletal muscle function after 6 week of bed rest. *J Appl Physiol, 82*, 182-188.

Bouhassira, D., Danziger, N., Atta, N. & Guirimand, F. (2003). Comparison of the pain suppressive effects of clinical and experimental painful conditioning stimuli. *Brain, 126*, 1068-1078.

Bozec, S. L., Evans, O. M. & Maton, B. (1987). Long-latency stretch reflexes of the human elbow extensors during voluntary relaxation: Differences between agonistic muscles. *Experimental Neurology, 96*, 516-527.

Brenner, B. & Yu, L. C. (1993). Structural changes in the actomyosin cross-bridges associated with force generation. *Procedings of National Academy of Sciences, 90*, 5252 - 5256.

Brooke, J. D., Cheng, J., Collins, D. F., Mcilroy, W. E., Misiaszek, J. E. & Stains, W. R. (1997). Sensori-sensory afferent conditioning with leg movement: Gain control in spinal reflex and ascending paths. *Progress in Neurology, 51*, 393-421.

Brooke, J. D., Mcilroy, W. E. & Collins, D. F. (1992). Movement features and H-reflex modulation. I. Pedalling versus matched controls. *Brain Research, 582*, 78-84.

Brooke, J. D., Mcilroy, W. E., Collins, D. F. & Misiaszek, J. E. (1995). Mechanisms within human spinal cord supress fast reflex to control the movement of the legs. *Brain Res, 679*, 255-260.

Brooke, M. H. & Kaplan, H. (1972). Muscle pathology in rheumatoid arthritis., polymyalgia rheumatica., and polymyositis: a histochemical study. *Arch Pathol, 94*, 101-118.

Brown, J. K., Rensburg, F. V. & Walsh, E. G. (1987). A neurological study of hand function of hemiplegic children. *Dev Med Child Neurol, 29*, 287-304.

Brown, T. I. H., Rack, P. M. H. & Ross, H. F. (1982). Electromyographic responses to imposed sinusoidal movement of the human thumb. *Journal of Physiology, 332*, 87-99.

Buchthal, F., Kaiser, E. & Rosenfalck, P. (1951). The rheology of the cross striated muscle fibre. *Dan Biol Medd, 21*, 1-318.

Burke, D., Andrews, C. J. & Gillies, J. D. (1971). The reflex response to sinusoidal stretching in spastic man. *Brain, 94*, 455-470.

Burks, K. & Keegan, K. (2006). Objective measurement of stiffness in knee osteoarthritis. *Orthopaedic Nursing, 25*, 244-250.

Burne, J. A., Hayes, M. W. & Yiannikas, C. (1995). Short-term fluctuations in Parkinsonian and essential tremor: reflex and central contributions. *Electroencephalography and Clinical Neurophysiology, 94*, 62.

Butler, D. L., Grood, E. S., Noyes, F. R. & Zernicke, R. F. (1978). *Bioemechanics of ligaments and tendons.*, 125-181.

Caccia, M. R., McComas, A. J., Upton, A. R. M. & Blogg, T. (1973). Cutaneous reflexes in small muscles of the hand. *Journal of Neurology, Neurosurgery and Psychiatry, 36*, 960-977.

Capaday, C. & Stein, R. B. (1986). Amplitude modulation of the soleus H-reflex in the human during walking and standing. *Journal of Neuroscience, 6*, 1308-1313.

Capaday, C. & Stein, R. B. (1987). Difference in the amplitude of the human soleus H-reflex during walking and running. *Journal of Physiology, 392*, 513-522.

Carter, R. R., Crago, P. E. & Gorman, P. H. (1993). Nonlinear stretch reflex interaction during cocontraction. *Journal of Neurophysiology, 69*, 943-952.

Carter, R. R., Crago, P. E. & Keith, M. W. (1990). Stiffness regulation by reflex action in the normal human hand. *Journal of Neurophysiology, 64*, 105-118.

Cathers, I., O'Dwyer, N. & Neilson, P. (1996). Tracking performance with sinusoidal and irregular targets under different conditions of peripheral feedback. *Experimental Brain Research, 111*, 437-446.

Cathers, I., O'Dwyer, N. & Neilson, P. (1999). Dependence of stretch reflexes on amplitude and bandwidth of stretch in human wrist muscle. *Experimental Brain Research, 129*, 278-287.

Cathers, I., O'Dwyer, N. & Neilson, P. (2004). Variation of magnitude and timing of wrist flexor stretch reflex across the full range of voluntary activation. *Experimental Brain Research, 157*, 324-335.

Chehata, J. C., Hassell, A. B., Clarke, S. A., Mattey, D. L., Jones, M. A., Jones P. W. & Dawes, P. T. (2001). Mortality in rheumatoid arthritis: relationship to single and composite measures of disease activity. *Rheumatology, 40*, 447 - 452.

Chen, R. & Ashby, P. (1993). Reflex responses in upper limb muscles to cutaneous stimuli. *Canadian Journal of Neurological Sciences, 20*, 271-278.

Choy, E. H. & Panayi, G. S. (2001). Cytokine pathways and joint inflammation in rheumatoid arthritis. *New England Journal of Medicine, 344*, 907-916.

Cody, F. W. J., Goodwin, C. N. & Richardson, H. C. (1987). Effects of ischaemia upon reflex electromyographic responses evoked by stretch and vibration in human wrist flexor muscles. *Journal of Physiology, 391*, 589-609.

Coggeshall, R. E., Hong, K. A. P., Langford, L. A., Schiable, H. G. & Schimidt, R. F. (1983). Discharge characteristic of fine medial articular afferents at rest and during passive movements of inflamed knee joints. *Brain Research, 272*, 185-188.

Crago, P. E., Houk, J. C. & Hasan, Z. (1976). Regulatory actions of human stretch reflex. *Journal of Neurophysiology, 39*, 925-935.

Curtiss, P. H. (1964). Changes produced in the synovial membrane and synovial fluid by disease. *Journal of Bone and Joint Surgery, 46*, 873-900.

Danneskiold-Samsoe, B. & Grimby, G. (1986a). Isokinetic and isometric muscle strength in patients with rheumatoid arthritis. The relationship to clinical parameters and the influence of corticosteroid. *Clin Rheumatol, 5*, 459-467.

Danneskiold-Samsoe, B. & Grimby, G. (1986b). The relationship between the leg muscle strength and physical capacity in patients with rheumatoid arthritis., with reference to the influence of corticosteroids. *Clin Rheumatol, 5*, 468-474.

de Palma, L., Chilleni, C., Albanelli, S., Rapali, S. & Beroni-Freddari, C. (2000). Muscle involvement in rheumatoid arthritis: an ultrastructural study. *Ultrastructural Pathology, 24*, 151-156.

deAndrade, J. R., Grant, C. & Dixon, A. J. (1965a). Joint distension and reflex muscle inhibition in the knee. *J Bone Joint Surg Am, 47*, 313-322.

Deandrade, J. R., Grant, C. & Dixon, A. S. (1965b). Joint Distension and Reflex Muscle Inhibition in the Knee. *Journal of Bone and Joint Surgery, 47*, 313-322.

DeBroucker, T. & al e., ed. (1989). *The nociceptive flexion reflex in humans: A specific and objective correlate of experimental pain*. Raven Press., Ltd., New York.

Doan, T. & Massarotti, E. (2005). Rheumatoid Arthritis: An overview of new and emerging therapies. *J Clin Pharmacol, 45*, 751-762.

Doemges, F. & Rack, P. M. H. (1992). Changes in the stretch reflex of the human first dorsal interosseus muscle during different tasks. *J Physiol, 447*, 563-573.

Dufresne, J. R., Soechting, J. F. & Terzuolo, C. A. (1980). Modulation of the myotactic reflex gain in man during intentional movement. *Brain Res, 193*, 67-84.

Duysens, J., Tax, A. A. M., Trippel, M. & Dietz, V. (1992). Phase-dependent reversal of reflexely induced movements during human gait. *Brain Res, 90*, 404-414.

Dyhre-Poulson, P., Simonsen, E. B. & Voigt, M. (1991). Dynamic control of muscle stiffness and H-reflex modulation during hopping and jumping in man. *J Physiol, 437*, 287-304.

Edamura, M., Yang, J. F. & Stein, R. B. (1991). Factors that determine the magnitude and time course of human H-reflexes in locomotion. *J Neurosci, 11*, 420-427.

Ekdahl, C. (1990). Muscle function in rheumatoid arthritis. Assessment and training. *Scandinavian Journal of Rheumatology supplement, 86*, 9-61.

Ekdahl, C., Andersson, S. I. & Svensson, B. (1989). Muscle function of the lower extremities in rheumatoid arthritis and osteoarthrosis. *Journal of Clinical Epidemiology, 42*.

Ekdahl, C. & Broman, G. (1992a). Muscle strength., endurance., and aerobic capacity in rheumatoid arthritis: a comparative study with healthy subjects. *Annals of Rheumatic Diseases, 51*, 35-40.

Ekdahl, C. & Broman, G. (1992b). Muscle strength., endurance., and aerobic capacity in rheumatoid arthritis: a comparative study with healthy subjects. *Annals of Rheumatic Diseases, 51*, 35-40.

Eklund, G. & Skoglund, S. (1960). On the specificity of the Ruffini like joint receptors. *Acta Physiologica Scandinavica, 49*, 184-191.

Emery, P. & Gibson, T. (1986). A double blind study of the simple analgesic nefopam in rheumatoid arthritis. *Br J Rheumatol, 25*, 72-76.

Escalante, A., Haas, R. W. & Rincon, I. (2005). A model of impairment and functional limitation in rheumatoid arthritis. *BMC Musculoskel Disord, 6*, 1-8.

Evans, A. L., Harrison, L. M. & Stephens, J. A. (1989). Task-dependent changes in cutaneous reflexes recorded from various muscles controlling finger movement in man. *Journal of Physiology, 418*, 1-12.

Fahrer, H., Rentsch, H. U., Gerber, N. J., Beyeler, C., Hess, C. W. & Grunig, B. (1988). Knee effusion and reflex inhibition of the quadriceps. A bar to effective retraining. *Journal of Bone and Joint Surgery (Br), 70*, 635-638.

Feldmann, M., Brennan, F. M. & Maini, R. N. (1996). Rheumatoid arthritis. *Cell, 85*, 307-310.

Fellows, S. J., Doemges, F., Topper, R., Thilmann, A. F. & Noth, J. (1993). Changes in the short and long latency stretch reflex components of the triceps surae muscle during ischemia in man. *J Physiol, 472*, 737-748.

Ferrell, W. R. (1980). The adequacy of stretch receptors in the cat knee joint for signalling joint angle throughout a full range of movement. *J Physiol, 299*, 85-100.

Finlay, J. B. (1978). Thixotropy in human skin. *J Biomech, 11*, 333-342.

Forsberg, H. (1979). Stumbling corrective reaction: a phase dependent compensatory reaction during locomotion. *J Neurophysiol, 42*, 936-953.

Fries, J. F., Spitz, P., Guy Kraines, R. & Holman, H. R. (1980). Measurement of patient outcome in arthritis. *Arthritis Rheum, 23*, 137-145.

Friewald, J., Reuter, I. & Engelhardt, M. ed. (1999). *Neuromuscular and motor system alterations after knee trauma and surgery.* Kluwer Academic/ Plenum Publishers., New York.

Gaffo, A., Saag, K. G. & Curtis, J. R. (2006). Treatment of rheumatoid arthritis. *American Journal of Health-System Pharmacology, 63*, 2451- 2465.

Geborek, P., Moritz, U. & Wollheim, F. A. (1989). Joint capsular stiffness in knee arthritis. Relationship to intraarticular volume., hydrostatic pressures., and extensor muscle function. *J Rheumatol, 16*, 1351-1358.

Goldblatt, F. & Isenberg, D. A. (2005). New therapies for rheumatoid arthritis. *Clinical and Experimental Immunology, 140*, 195-204.

Gollhofer, A., Schopp, A., Rapp, W. & Stroinik, V. (1998). Changes in reflex excitability following isometric contraction in humans. *Eur J Appl Physiol, 77*, 89-97.

Gordon, J. & Ghez, C. ed. (1991). *Muscle receptors and spinal reflexes: The stretch reflex.* Appleton and Lange. Norwalk.

Gottlieb, G. L. & Agarwal, G. C. (1979). Response to sudden torques about ankle in man: Myotatic reflex. *J Neurophysiol, 42*, 91-106.

Hagbarth, K. E., Hagglund, J. V., Nordin, M. & Wallin, E. U. (1985). Thixotropic behaviour of human finger flexor muscles with accompanying changes in spindle and reflex responses to stretch. *J Physiol, 368*, 323-342.

Haigh, R. C., McCabe, C. S., Halligan, P. W. & Blake, D. R. (2003). Joint stiffness in a phantom limb: evidence of central nervous system involvement in rheumatoid arthritis. *Rheumatology (Oxford), 42*, 888-892.

Hakkinen, A., Hannonen, P. & Hakkinen, K. (1995). Muscle strength in healthy people and in patients suffering from recent-onset inflammatory arthritis. *Br J Rheumatol, 34*, 355-360.

Halkjaer-Kristensen, J. & Ingemann-Hansen, T. (1985). Wasting of the human quadriceps muscle after knee ligament injuries. *Scandinavian Journal of Rehabilitaion Medicine, 13*, 5-55.

Halla, J. T., Koopman, W. J., Fallahi, S., Oh, S. J., Gay, R. E. & Schrohenloher, R. E. (1984). Rheumatoid myositis. Clinical and histologic features and possible pathogenesis. *Arthritis and Rheumatism, 27*, 737-743.

Harvey, A. R. (1987). Neurophysiology of rheumatic pain. *Clinical Rheumatology, 1.*

Harvey, L., Herbert, R. D. & Crosbie, J. (2002). Does stretching induce lasting increases in joint ROM? A systemic review. *Physiotherapy Research International, 7*, 1-13.

Hasan, Z. & Stuart, D. G. ed. (1984). Mammalian muslce receptors., *vol. 3: Anatomy and Physiology.* Marcel Decker., New York.

Hassan, B. S., Doherty, S. A., Mockett, S. & Doherty, M. (2002). Effect of pain reduction on postural sway., proprioception and quadriceps strength in subjects with knee osteoarthritis. *Annals of Rheumatic Diseases, 61*, 422-428.

Hassan, B. S., Mockett, S. & Doherty, S. A. (2001). Static postural sway., proprioception., and maximal voluntary quadriceps contraction in patients with knee osteoarthtitis and normal control subjects. *Annals of Rheumatic Diseases, 60*, 612-618.

Hazes, J. M. W., Hayton, R. & Silman, A. J. (1993). A reevaluation of the symptom of morning stiffness. *J Rheumatol, 20*, 1138-1142.

Heerkens, Y. F., Woittiez, R. D. & Huijing, P. A. (1986). Passive resistance of the human knee the effect of immobilization. *J Biomech Eng, 8*, 95-105.

Heerkens, Y. F., Woittiez, R. D. & Huijing, P. A. (1987). Passive resistance of the human knee the effect of re-mobilization. *J Biomech Eng, 9*, 69-76.

Helliwell, P. S. (1994). Normal vibration perception thresholds in rheumatoid arthritis- Evidence against the neurogenic theory of articular stiffness. *Clin Rheumatol, 13*, 51-53.

Helliwell, P. S. (1995). The semiology of arthritis: Discriminating between patients on the basis of their symptoms. *Annals of Rheumatic Diseases, 54*, 924-926.

Helliwell, P. S. (1997). Use of an objective measure of articular stiffness to record changes in finger joints after intra-articular injection of corticosteroid. *Ann Rheum Dis, 56*, 71-73.

Helliwell, P. S., Howe, A. & Wright, V. (1987a). Functional assessment of the hand; acceptability., reproducibility and utility of a new system for measuring strength. *Ann Rheum Dis, 46*, 203-208.

Helliwell, P. S., Howe, A. & Wright, V. (1987b). The measurement of stiffness in rheumatoid hand. *Eng Med, 16*, 203-207.

Helliwell, P. S., Howe, A. & Wright, V. (1988). Lack of objective evidence of stiffness in rheumatoid arthritis. *Ann Rheum Dis, 47*, 754-758.

Helliwell, P. S. & Jackson, S. (1994). Relationship between weakness and muscle wasting in rheumatoid arthritis. *Annals of Rheumatic Diseases, 53*, 726-728.

Herbison, G. J., Jaweed, M. M. & Ditunno, J. F. (1979). Muscle atrophy in rats following denervation., casting., inflammation., and tenotomy. *Archives of Physiology and Medical Rehabilitation, 60*, 401-404.

Hill, D. K. (1968). Tension due to interaction between the sliding filaments in resting striated muscle. The effect of stimulation. *J Physiol, 199*, 637-684.

Hoffer, J. A. & Andreassen, S. (1981). Regulation of soleus muscle stiffness in premammillary cats: intrinsic and reflex components. *J Neurophysiol, 45*, 267-285.

Hopkins, J. T. & Ingersoll, C. D. (2000). Arthrogenic muscle inhibition: A limiting factor in joint rehabilitation. *Journal of Sports Rehabilitation, 9*, 135-159.

Hopkins, J. T., Ingersoll, C. D. & Edwards, J. E. (2002). Cryotherapy and TENS decrease arthrogenic muscle inhibition of the vastus medialis following knee joint effusion. *Journal of Athletic Training, 37*, 25-32.

Hopkins, J. T., Ingersoll, C. D. & Krause, B. A. (2001). Effect of knee joint effusion on quadriceps and soleus motoneuron pool excitability. *Med Sci Sports Excercise, 33*, 123-126.

Houk, J. C. (1979). Regulation of stiffness by skeletomotor reflexes. *Annu Rev Physiol, 41*, 99-114.

Houk, J. C. & Rymer, W. Z. ed. (1981). *Neural control of muscle length and tension.*, vol. II., Motor Control. American Physiological Society., Bethesda.

Hsieh, L. F., Didenko, B., Schumacher, H. R., Jr. & Torg, J. S. (1987). Isokinetic and isometric testing of knee musculature in patients with rheumatoid arthritis with mild knee involvement. *Archives of Physiology and Medical Rehabilitation, 68*, 294-297.

Hufschimidt, A. & Schwaller, I. (1987). Short-range elasticity and resting tension of relaxed human lower leg muscles. *J Physiol, 391*, 451-465.

Hugon, M., ed. (1973). *Exteroceptive reflexes to stimulation of sural nerve in man.*, vol. 3. Karger., Basel.

Hunter, I. W. & Kearney, R. E. (1982). Dynamics of human ankle stiffness: variation with mean ankle torque. *J Biomech, 15*, 747-752.

Hurley, M. V. & Newham, D. J. (1993). The influence of arthrogenous muscle inhibition on quadriceps rehabilitaion of patients with early., unilateral osteoarthritic knees. *Br J Rheumatol, 32*, 127-131.

Iles, J. F., Stokes, M. & Young, A. (1990). Reflex actions of knee joint afferents during contraction of the human quadriceps. *Clin Physiol, 10*, 489-500.

Ingersoll, C. D., Palmieri, R. M. & Hopkins, J. T. (2003). A joint dilemma. In *The Interdisciplinary Journal of Rehabilitation*. Los Angeles.

Jenner, J. R. & Stephens, J. A. (1982). Cutaneous reflex responses and their central nervous pathways studied in man. *Journal of Physiology, 333*, 405-419.

Johansson, H. & Sojka, P. (1991). Pathophysiological mechanisms involved in genesis and spread of muscular tension in occupational muscle pain and in chronic musculoskeletal pain syndromes: A hypothesis. *Medical Hypothesis, 35*, 196-203.

Johns, R. J. & Wright, V. (1962). Relative importance of various tissues in joint stiffness. *J Appl Physiol, 17*, 824-828.

Johnson, M. T. V., Kipnis, A. N., Lee, M. C. & Loewenson, R. B. (1991). Modulation of the stretch reflex during volitional sinusoidal tracking in Parkinson's disease. *Brain, 114*, 443-460.

Joyce, G. C., Rack, P. M. H. & Ross, H. F. (1974). The forces generated at the human elbow joint in response to imposed sinusoidal movements of the forearm. *J Physiol, 240*, 351-374.

Kearney, R. E. & Hunter, I. W. (1982). Dynamics of human ankle stiffness: variation with displacement amplitude. *J Biomech, 15*, 753-756.

Kearney, R. E., Stein, R. B. & Parameswaran, L. (1997). Identification of intrinsic and reflex contributions to human ankle stiffness dynamics. *IEEE Trans Biomed Eng, 44*, 493-504.

Kellgren, J. H. & Lawrence, J. S. (1957). Radiological ssesment of osteo-arthrosis. *Annals of the Rheumatic Diseases, 16*, 494 - 502.

Kennedy, J. C., Alexander, I. J. & Hayes, K. C. (1982). Nerve supply of the human knee and its functional importance. *Am J Sports Med, 10*, 329-335.

Kimura, T., Nozaki, D., Nakazawa, K., Akai, M. & Ohtsuki, T. (2003). Gradual increment/decrement of isometric force modulates soleus strech reflex response in humans. *Neurosci Lett, 347*, 25-28.

Kirsch, R. F., Boskov, D. & Rymer, W. Z. (1994a). Muscle stiffness during transient and continuous movements of cat muscle: Perturbation characteristics and physiological relevance. *IEEE Trans Biomed Eng, 41*, 758-770.

Kirsch, R. F. & Kearney, R. E. (1997). Identification of time-varying stiffness dynamics of the human ankle joint during an imposed movement. *Exp Brain Res, 114*, 71-85.

Kirsch, R. F., Kearney, R. E. & Crago, P. E. (1994b). Dynamic stiffness measurement and the control of movement. *IEEE Trans Biomed Eng*, 428-429.

Kirsch, R. F., Kearney, R. E. & MacNeil, J. B. (1993). Identification of time varying dynamics of the human triceps surae stretch reflex: I Rapid isometric contraction. *Experimental Brain Research, 97*, 115-127.

Kleinbohl, D., Trojan, J., Konrad, C. & Holzl, R. (2006). Sensitization and habituation of AMH and C-fiber related percepts of repetitive radiant heat stimulation. *Clinical Neurophysiology, 117*, 118-130.

Klepper, S. E. (2003). Exercise and fitness in children with arthritis: Evidence of benefits for exercise and physical activity. *Arthritis Rheum, 49*, 435-443.

Kniffki, K. D., Mense, S. & Schmidt, R. F. (1978). Responses of Group IV afferent units from skeletal muscle to stretch., contraction and chemical stimulation. *Experimental Brain Research, 31*, 511-522.

Koltzenburg, M., Torebjork, H. E. & Wahren, L. K. (1994). Nociceptor modulated central sensitization causes mechanical hyperalgesia in acute chemogenic and chronic neuropathic pain. *Brain, 117*, 579-591.

Lakie, M. & Robson, L. G. (1988b). Thixotropy: Stiffness recovery rate in relaxed frog muscle. *Exp Physiol, 73*, 237-239.

Lakie, M., Walsh, E. G. & Wright, G. W. (1984). Resonance at the wrist demonstrated by the use of a torque motor: An instrumental analysis of muscle tone in man. *J Physiol, 353*, 265-285.

Lamontagne, A., Malouin, F., Richards, C. L. & Dumas, F. (1998). Evaluation of reflex and nonreflex induced muscle resistance to stretch in adults with spinal cord injury using hand-held and isokinetic dynamometry. *Physical Therapy, 78*, 964-978.

Lang, A. H., Kalliomaki, J. L., Puusa, A. & Halonen, J. P. (1981). Sensory neuropathy in rheumatoid arthritis: an electroneurographic study. *Scand J Rheumatol, 10*, 81-84.

Lansbury, J. (1958). Report of a three-year study on the systemic and articular indexes in rheumatoid arthritis *Arthritis and Rheumatism, 1*, 505.

Lanzillo, B., Pappone, N., Crisci, C., di Girolamo, C., Massini, R. & Caruso, G. (1998). Subclinical peripheral nerve involvement in patients with rheumatoid arthritis. *Arhtritis and Rheumatism, 41*, 1196-1202.

LaRoche, D. P. & Connolly, D. A. J. (2006). Effects of stretching on passive muscle tension and response to eccentric exercise. *Am J Sports Med, 34*, 1000-1007.

Latash, M. L. (1993). *Control of human movement*. Human Kinetics Publishers., Chicago., IL.

Lee, D. M. & Weinblatt, M. E. (2001). Rheumatoid arthritis. *Lancet, 358*, 903-911.

Lee, R. G. & Tatton, W. G. ed. (1978). *Long loop reflexes in man.*, vol. 4. Karger., Basel.

Lin, F. M. & Sabbahi, M. (1998). The aging effects on the EMG and mechanical responses of the human wrist flexor stretch reflexes. *Electromyogr Clin Neurophysiol, 38*.

Lindehammar, H. & Lindvall, B. (2004). Muscle involvement in juvenile idiopathic arthritis. *Rheumatology (Oxford), 43*, 1546-1554.

Lineker, S., Badley, E., Charles, C., Hart, L. & Streiner, D. (1999). Defining morning stiffness in rheumatoid arthritis. *J Rheumatol, 26*, 1052-1057.

Linke, W. A. (2000). Titin elasticity in the context of the sarcomere: force and extensibility measurements on single myofibrils. *Adv Exp Med Biol, 481*, 179-202.

Loeser, J. D. (2000). *Ablative neurosurgical operations - introduction*. Lippincott, Philadelphia.

Lundberg, A., Malmgren, K. & Schomburg, E. D. (1978). Role of joint afferents in motor control exemplfied by effects on reflex pathways from Ib afferents. *J Physiol, 284*, 327-343.

Luqmani, R., Hennell, S. & Estrach, C. (2006). British Society for Rheumatology and British Health Professionals in Rheumatology Guideline for the Management of Rheumatoid Arthritis (the first two years). *Rheumatology (Oxford), 45*, 1167-1169.

Magyar, E., Talerman, A., Mohacsy, J., Wouters, H. W. & de Buijn, W. C. (1977). Muscle changes in rheumatoid arthritis. *Virchows Archives, A Pathological Anatomy and Histology, 373*, 267-278.

Mah, C. D. (2001). Spatial and temporal modulation of joint stiffness during multijoint movement. *Exp Brain Res, 136*, 492-506.

Marsden, C. D., Merton, P. A. & Morton, H. B. (1972). Servo action in human voluntary movement. *Nature, 238*, 140-143.

Marsden, C. D., Merton, P. A. & Morton, H. B. (1974). Behaviour of short and long latency components of the stretch reflex in human muscle. *Proceedings of the Physiological Society*, 43-44.

Marsden, C. D., Merton, P. A. & Morton, H. B. (1976). Stretch reflex and servo action in a variety of human muscles. *J Physiol, 259*, 531-560.

Marsden, C. D., Merton, P. A., Morton, H. B., Adam, J. E. R. & Hallett, M., ed. (1978). *Automatic and voluntary responses to muscle stretch in man.*, vol. 4. Karger., Basel.

Matre, D. A., Sinkjaer, T., Svensson, B. P. & Nielson, L. N. (1998). Experimental muscle pain increases the human stretch reflex. *Pain, 75*, 331-339.

Matthews, P. B. C. (1984). Evidence from the use of vibration that the human long-latency stretch reflex depends upon spindle secondary afferents. *J Physiol, 348*, 383-415.

Matthews, P. B. C. (1989). Long-latency stretch reflexes of two intrinsic muscles of the human hand analysed by cooling the arm. *J Physiol, 419*, 519-538.

Matthews, P. B. C. (1993). Interaction between short- and long-latency components of the human stretch reflex during sinusoidal stretching. *J Physiol, 462*, 503-527.

Matthews, P. B. C. & Stein, R. B. (1969). The sensitivity of muscle spindle afferents to small sinusoidal changes of length. *J Physiol, 200*, 723-743.

McCrea, D. A. (2001). Spinal circuitry of sensorimotor control of locomotion. *J Physiol, 533*, 41-50.

Mcilroy, W. E., Collins, D. F. & Brooke, J. D. (1992). Movement features and H-reflex modulation. II Passive rotation., movement velocity and single leg movement. *Brain Res, 582*, 85-93.

McMahon, S. & Koltzenburg, M. (1990). The changing role of primary afferent neurones in pain. *Pain, 43*, 269-272.

Menadue, C., Raymond, J., Kilbreath, S. L., Refshauge, K. M. & Adams, R. (2006). *Reliability of two goniometric methods of measuring active inversion and eversion range of motion at the ankle.*, vol. 7.

Merton, P. A. (1953). *Speculations on the servo control of movement.* Little Brown., Boston.

Mills, K. (1970). Pathology of the knee joint in rheumatoid arthritis. *J Bone Joint Surg Am, 52*, 746-756.

Milner, T. E. (1993). Dependence of elbow viscoelastic behaviour on speed and loading in voluntary movements. *Exp Brain Res, 93*, 177-180.

Minajeva, A., Kulke, M., Fernandez, J. M. & Linke, W. A. (2001). Unfolding of titin domains explains the viscoelastic behaviour of skeletal myofibrils. *Journal of Biophysics, 80*, 1442-1451.

Mirbagheri, M. M., Barbeau, H. & Kearney, R. E. (2000). Intrinsic and reflex contributions to human ankle stiffness: variation with activation level and position. *Exp Brain Res, 135*, 423-436.

Miro, O., Pedrol, E. & Casademont, J. (1996). Muscle involvement in rheumatoid arthritis: clinicopathological study of 21 symptomatic cases. *Seminars in Arthritis and Rheumatism, 25*, 421-428.

Moreland, L. W. (1999). Inhibitors of tumor necrosis factor: new treatment options for rheumatoid arthritis. *Cleveland Clinical Journal of Medicine, 66*, 367-374.

Nakamura, T., Kurosawa, H., Kawahara, H., Watarai, K. & Miyashita, H. (1986). Muscle fiber atrophy in the quadriceps in knee-joint disorders. Histochemical studies on 112 cases. *Archives of Orthopedic Trauma and Surgery, 105*, 163-169.

Nakazawa, K., Yamamoto, S. I. & Yano, H. (1997). Short- and long-latency reflex responses during different motor tasks in elbow flexor muscles. *Exp Brain Res, 116*, 20-28.

Neilson, P. D. (1972). Interaction between voluntary contraction and tonic stretch reflex transmission in normal and spastic patients. *J Neurol Neurosurg Psychiatry, 35*, 853-860.

Neilson, P. D. (1973). Effect of procaine infiltration into biceps brachii muscle in man on supraspinal control of reflex transmission. *J Neurol Neurosurg Psychiatry, 36*, 87-93.

Neilson, P. D., ed. (1993). *Tonic stretch reflex in normal subjects and in cerebral palsy.* Cambridge Univerisity Press., Cambridge.

Neilson, P. D. & Neilson, M. D. (1978). The role of action reflexes in the damping of mechanical oscillations. *Brain Res, 142*, 439-453.

Nichols, T. R. & Houk, J. C. (1976). Improvement in linearity and regulation of stiffness that results from actions of stretch reflex. *J Neurophysiol, 29*, 119-142.

Noth, J., Schwarz, M., Podoll, K. & Montamedi, F. (1991). Evidence that low-threshold muscle afferents evoke long-latency stretch reflexes in human hand muscles. *J Neurophysiol, 65*, 1089-1097.

O'Reilly, S. C., Jones, A., Muir, K. R. & Doherty, M. (1998). Quadriceps weakness in knee osteoarthritis: the effect on pain and disability. *Annals of Rheumatic Diseases, 57*, 588-594.

Oatis, C. A., Adonizio, M. A., Gillum, J. B. & Kousen, C. L. (1995). Knee joint stiffness in subjects with osteoarthritis versus healthy subjects. *Arthritis Rheum, 38*, S153.

Price, D. D. (2002). Central neural mechanisms that interrelate sensory and affective dimensions of pain. *Molecular Interventions, 2*, 392-402.

Proske, U., Morgan, D. L. & Gregory, J. E. (1993). Thixotropy in skeletal muscle and in muscle spindles. *Prog Neurobiol, 41*, 705-721.

Purslow, P. P. (1989). Strain-induced reorientation of an intramuscular connective tissue network: implications for passive muscle elasticity. *J Biomech, 22*, 21-31.

Rack, P. M. H. (1981). Limitations of somatosensory feedback in control of posture and movement. In *Handbook of Physiology: The nervous system.*, ed. Geiger SR., 229-256. American Physiological Society., Bethesda.

Rack, P. M. H., Ross, H. F. & Brown, T. I. H., ed. (1978). *Reflex responses during sinusoidal movement in human limbs.*, vol. 4. Progress in Clinical Neurophysiology., Karger., Basel.

Rack, P. M. H., Ross, H. F., Thilmann, A. F. & Walters, D. K. W. (1983). Reflex responses at the human ankle: the importance of tendon compliance. *J Physiol, 344*, 503-524.

Rack, P. M. H. & Westbury, D. R. (1974). The short range stiffness of active mamalian muscle and its effect on mechanical properties. *J Physiol, 240*, 331-350.

Rajagopalan, A. & Burne, J. (2010). Stretch reflexes and joint dynamics in rheumatoid arthritis. *Exp Brain Res, 201*, 37-45.

Rasker, J. J., Peters, H. J. G. & Boon, K. L. (1986). Influence of weather on stiffness and force in patients with rheumatoid arthritis. *Scand J Rheumatol, 15*, 27-36.

Riemann, B. L. & Lephart, S. M. (2002). The sensorimotor system., Part II: The role of proprioception in motor control and functional joint stability. *Journal of Athletic Training, 37*, 80-84.

Roush, J. R., Bustillo, K. & Low, E. (2008). Measurement error between a goniometer and the NIH ImageJ program for measuring quadriceps angle. In *The Internet Journal of Allied Health Sciences and Practice*.

Sandkuhler, J. & Liu, X. (1998). Induction of long-term potentiation at spinal synapses by noxious stimulation or nerve injury. *European Journal of Neuroscience, 10*, 2476-2480.

Schaible, H. G., Neugebaur, V., Cervero, F. & Schmidt, R. F. (1991). Changes in tonic descending inhibition of of spinal neurons with articular input during the development of acute arthritis in the cat. *J Neurophysiol, 66*, 1021-1032.

Scot, J. T. (1960). Diurnal variation in grip strength. *Annals of Rheumatic Diseases, 19*, 362-368.

Shakespeare, D. T. (1985). Reflex inhibition of the quadriceps after meniscectomy: Lack of association with pain. *Clin Physiol, 5*, 137-144.

Siddiqui, M. A. A. (2007). The efficacy and tolerability of newer biologics in rheumatoid arthritis: best current evidence. *Current Opinion in Rheumatology, 19*, 308-313.

Sinkjaer, T. & Hayashi, R. (1989). Regulation of wrist stiffness by the stretch reflex. *J Biomech, 22*, 1133-1140.

Sinkjaer, T. & Magnussen, I. (1994). Passive intrinsic and reflex-mediated stiffness in the ankle extensors of hemiparetic patients. *Brain, 117*, 355-363.

Sinkjaer, T., Toft, E., Larsen, K., Andreassen, S. & Hansen, H. J. (1993). Non-reflex and reflex mediated ankle joint stiffness in multiple sclerosis patients with spasticity. *Muscle Nerve, 16*, 69-76.

Sivri, A. & Guler-Uysal, F. (1998). The electroneurophysiological evaluation of rheumatoid arthritis patients. *Clin Rheumatol, 17*, 416-418.

Slemenda, C., Brandt, K. D. & Heilman, D. K. (1997). Quadriceps weakness and osteoarthritis of the knee. *Ann Intern Med, 127*, 97-104.

Smolen, J. S., Aletaha, D., Koeller, M., Weisman, M. H. & Emery, P. (2007). New therapies for treatment of rheumatoid arthritis. *Lancet, 370*, 1861-1874.

Stam, J. & van Creval, H. (1989). Measurement of tendon reflexes by surface electromyography in normal subjects. *J Neurol, 236*, 231-237.

Staud, R., Vierck, C. J., Cannon, R. L., Mauderli, A. P. & Price, D. D. (2001). Abnormal sensitization and temporal summation of second pain (wind-up) in patients with fibromyalgia syndrome. *Pain, 91*, 165-175.

Stein, R. B. (1995). Presynaptic inhibition in humans. *Prog Neurobiol, 47*, 533-544.

Stein, R. B. & Capaday, C. (1988). The modulation of human reflexes during functional motor tasks. *TINS, 11*, 328-332.

Stein, R. B., French, A. S. & Holden, A. V. (1972). The frequency response., coherence., and information capacity of two neuronal models. *Biophys J, 12*, 295-322.

Stein, R. B. & Kearney, R. E. (1995). Nonlinear behaviour of muscle reflexes at the human ankle joint. *J Neurophysiol, 73*, 65-72.

Steinberg, V. L. & Wynn-Parry, C. B. (1961). Electromyographic changes in rheumatoid arthritis. *Br Med J, 1*, 630-632.

Stenstrom, C. H. & Minor, M. A. (2003). Evidence for the benefit of aerobic and strengthening exercise in rheumatoid arthritis. *Arthritis Rheum, 49*, 428-434.

Stokes, M. & Young, A. (1984). The contribution of reflex inhibition to arthrogenous muscle weakness. *Clinical Science, 67*, 7-14.

Stucki, G., Bruhlmann, P., Stucki, S. & Michel, B. A. (1998). Isometric muscle strength is an indicator of self-reported physical functional disability in patients with rheumatoid arthritis. *Br J Rheumatol, 37*, 643-648.

Thilmann, A. F., Schwarz, M., Toppper, R., Fellows, S. J. & Noth, J. (1991). Different mechanisms underlie the long-latency stretch reflex response of active human muscle at different joints. *J Physiol, 444*, 631-643.

Thompson, D. T., Wright, V. & Dowson, D. (1978). A new form of knee arthrograph for the study of stiffness. *Eng Med, 7*, 492.

Toft, E., Sinkjaer, T. & Andreassen, S. (1989). Mechanical and electromyographic responses to stretch of the human anterior tibial muscle at different levels of contraction. *Exp Brain Res, 74*, 213-219.

Unsworth, A., Bey, P. M. A. & Haslock, I. (1981). Stiffness in the metacarpo-phalangeal joints of young adults. *Clin Phys Physiol Meas, 2*, 123-133.

Unsworth, A., Yung, P. & Haslock, I. (1982). Measurement of stiffness in metacarpophalangeal joint: the arthrograph. *Clin Phys Physiol Meas, 3*, 273-281.

Valle, M. S., Casabona, A., Sgarlata, R., Garozzo, R., Vinci, M. & Cioni, M. (2006). The pendulum test as a tool to evaluate passive knee stiffness and viscosity of patients with rheumatoid arthritis. *BMC Musculoskel Disord, 7*, 89.

Vattanasilp, W., Ada, L. & Crosbie, J. (2000). Contribution of thixotropy., spasticity and contracture to ankle stiffness after stroke. *J Neurol Neurosurg Psychiatry, 69*, 34-39.

Walsh, E. G. (1992a). *Muscles, masses amd motion*. Mac Keith Press., Oxford.

Walsh, E. G. (1992b). Postural thixotropy: a significant factor in the stiffness of paralysed limbs? *Paraplegia, 30*, 113 - 115.

Wartenburg, R. (1951). Pendulousness of the leg as a diagnostic test. *Neurology, 1*, 18-24.

Weiss, P. L., Hunter, I. W. & Kearney, R. E. (1988). Human ankle joint stiffness over the full range of muscle activation levels. *J Biomech, 21*, 539-544.

Weiss, P. L., Kearney, R. E. & Hunter, I. W. (1986). Position dependence of stretch reflex dynamics at the human ankle. *Exp Brain Res, 63*, 49-59.

Wendler, J., Hummel, T., Reissinger, M., Manger, B., Pauli, E., Kalden, J. R. & Kobal, G. (2001). Patients with rheumatoid arthritis adapt differently to repetitive painful stimuli compared to healthy controls. *Journal of Clinical Neuroscience, 8*, 272-277.

Wessel, J. (1996). Isometric strength measurements of knee extensors in women with osteoarthritis of the knee. *J Rheumatol, 23*, 328-331.

Willer, J. C. (1977). Comparative study of perceived pain and nociceptive flexion reflex in man. *Pain, 3*, 69-80.

Willer, J. C., ed. (1984). *Nociceptive flexion reflex as a physiological correlate of pain sensation in humans*. Elsevier Science Publishers., Amsterdam.

Winkelstein, B. A. (2004). Mechanisms of central sensitization., neuroimmunology and injury biomechanics in persistent pain: implications for musculoskeletal disorders. *Journal of Elecromyography and Kinesiology, 14*, 87-93.

Wright, V. (1959). Some observations on diurnal variation of grip. *Clinical Science, 18*, 17.

Wright, V. & Johns, R. J. (1960a). Physical factors concerned with the stiffness of normal and diseased joints. *Bulletin of the Johns Hopkins Hospital, 106*, 215-231.

Wright, V. & Johns, R. J. (1960b). Observations on the measurement of joint stiffness. *Arhtritis and Rheumatism, 3*, 328-340.

Wright, V. & Johns, R. J. (1961). Quantitative and qualitative analysis of joint stiffness in normal subjects and in patients with connective tissue diseases. *Ann Rheum Dis, 20*, 36-45.

Xia, R., Bush, B. M. H. & Karst, G. M. (2005). Phase-dependent and task-dependent modulation of stretch reflexes during rhythmical hand tasks in humans. *J Physiol, 5643*, 941-951.

Young, A. (1993). Current issues in arthrogenous inhibition. *Annals of Rheumatic Diseases, 52*, 829-834.

Zehr, E. P. & Chua, R. (2000). Modulation of human cutaneous reflexes during rhythmic cyclical arm movement. *Experimental Brain Research, 135*, 241-250.

Zehr, E. P., Hesketh, K. L. & Chua, R. (2001). Differential regulation of cutaneous and H-reflexes during leg cycling in humans. *Journal of Neurophysiology, 85*, 1178-1184.

Zehr, E. P. & Stein, R. B. (1999). What functions do reflexes serve during human locomotion. *Prog Neurobiol, 58*, 185-205.

Zvaifler, N. J. (1973). The immunopathology of joint inflammation in rheumatoid arthritis. *Advances in Immunology, 16*, 265-336.

In: Rheumatoid Arthritis: Prevalence, Risk...
Editor: Michael H. Madsen

ISBN: 978-1-61761-931-1

Chapter 3

Hand Involvement and Its Effects on Quality of Life in Rheumatoid Arthritis

Nilay Sahin [*] ***and Hatice Ugurlu***
Selcuk University, Meram Faculty of Medicine, Physical Medicine and Rehabilitation Department, Meram/Konya, Turkey

Abstract

Rheumatoid arthritis (RA) is a chronic, inflammatory, progressive and systemic disease. Hand and wrist are the first involved parts in RA and this situation seriously affects the hand functions. Hand functions are quite important in daily living activities. Hand involvement and hand functions, are the major determinant of the course of disease and important cause of RA related disabilities. Problems in rheumatoid hand seen in different types. It is possible to classify the problems according to manifestation, anatomical parts or pathological conditions. In order to be successful in rheumatoid hand therapy it is important to understand the pathogenesis of the problem. Basically, after the pathological stages such as, tenosynovitis, tendon rupture, edema, subluxation, laxity, nodule development, contracture, functional uses of hand is limited. Early recognizing and treatment of problems in hand will increase the life quality of patient. Because lesions in RA are progressive and deformities develops during disease period. So, which methods will be helpful for doctors in diagnosis of these processes in early period? What is the position of physical examination in this methods. Besides of assessment of mentioned pathologies one by one, hand functions should be assessed globally. Many indicators been developed for this. But it is important to note that the clinic uses of these indicators are not practical and seems the differences in personal, professional and social necessities of individuals. Basically, it is very important to observe the patient continuous, to keep the deformity at minimum level and prevent them without new

[*] Corresponding author: Selcuk University, Meram Faculty of Medicine, Physical Medicine and Rehabilitation Department, Meram/Konya, Turkey, email: nilaysahin@gmail.com], tel: +90 5552332535 fax:+90 2126766200

formations during the RA treatment. There are several types of treatment including different multidisciplinary approaches for every problem.

Introduction

Rheumatoid arthritis (RA) is a chronic, systemic, inflammatory disease which involves the joint as well as the synovial tissue, causes progressive joint destruction and disability [1]. The clinical course of the disease can be anywhere between a mild, self-limited arthritis picture to a progressive multi-system involvement. In general the basic problem is the joint damage. It especially affects the wrist and the smaller joints of the hand. The hand and the wrist involvements are observed in 80% to 90% of RA cases [2]. For this reason during the examination, clinicians initially evaluate the hands and wrists of the patients with RA. Directly affecting the hand functions, the hand and wrist involvements are the most critical factors defining the daily activities and causing disabilities related to RA [3, 4]. Different forms of hand disabilities are noted for more than 70% of the patients with RA [3]. In order for the hand to be used efficiently; anatomical integrity, range of motion (ROM), muscle strength, coordination and sensation should be normal; also, there shouldn't be any pain [3, 5]. For the patients with RA, in early periods the joint damages in the hand and wrist disrupt the function of hand, but this condition is tried to be compensated with adaptation mechanisms [6]. To cope with developing the hand problems during the RA first the pathogenesis of deformity should be understood.

Pathogenesis

The primary targets of this disease are the tendons and synovium; and the secondary targets are periarticular tissue, muscles and blood vessels. Cellular hyperplasia and inflammatory reaction increased with angiogenesis form the basic pathogenesis of RA in cellular level. When synovium gets proliferous and hypertrophic, it causes articular cartilage destruction, subchondral bone invasion with the enzymatic reactions and changes on the surrounding tissue by stretching the soft tissues [7, 8].

The proliferative phase of the beginning is characterized by pain with movement, limited ability of movement, swelling causing compression of nerves and accumulation of fibrin. Phenomenon starts first in the synovial membrane. The proliferation of the synoviocytes that remind macrophage and fibroblasts causes a thickening of the synovial membrane. Angiogenesis accompany synovial proliferation in order to support new growth and to allow the leucocytic infiltration. Besides these cells, T cells, B cells, mast cells and plasma cells infiltrate to synovial area and lead to pannus development. With the current knowledge it is argued that T cells have an important place in this phase [9].

Pannus which is the consequence of constant cell invasion of the synovial membrane causes erosion in the bone and cartilage particularly by preventing the nutrition of the cartilage. In addition to this, the villose formation in the synovium causes stretching of the ligaments and capsules by causing effusion at the joints. Thereby the destructive phase, where the instabilities and deformations develop at the joints and tendon ruptures occur, starts.

During this phase, there is a high amount of pro-inflammatory cytokines and the metalloproteinase which accompany them in the environment. Tumor necrosis factor-alpha and interleukin-1 are the two main cytokines in the environment [7, 8].

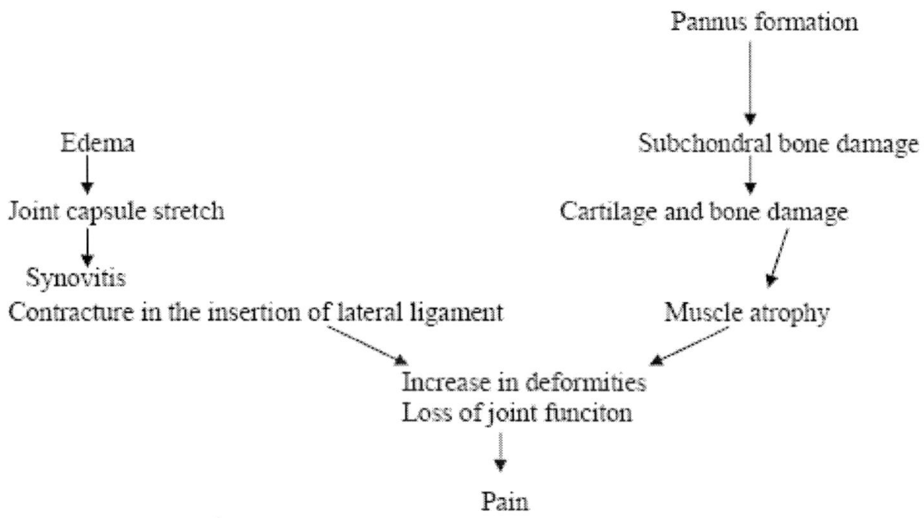

Figure 1. The pathogenesis of deformities in rheumatoid arthritis

At the last phase inflammatory reaction comes to an end and tendon adhesions and fibrosis which causes permanent deformations start [8] (Figure 1). As a result, the pathological period which takes place at the hand and wrist joints of the RA patient causes pain, instability and deformity, therefore interference with the hand functions. Problems occurring at the rheumatoid hand can be analyzed with Hasting classification, which is made according to the deformations of the hand, joint involvement and tendon involvement [8]. It can also be analyzed by the classification according to pathogenesis. In the classification according to the pathological picture, the hand-wrist problems can be analyzed under 5 main titles:

1) Tendinitis and tenosynovitis
2) Tendon rupture
3) Deformity and subluxation
4) Entrapment neuropathy
5) Nodules

1) Tendinitis-Tenosynovitis

Tendons are consistent, steady collagen bunches attached tightly to each other, elongated cylindrical structures formed in the amorphous connective tissues between these bunches and anatomical regions attached to muscles. This structure is surrounded by the loose connective tissue which carries the blood vessels and nerves. Its basic role is to limit excessive stretching of the tendon fibers and muscle tonus. The concentric and excentric contractions of the muscles provide the daily activities by creating adequate elongations and tensions on the tendon fibers [10, 11].

The tendon involvement can be seen in RA and as a result of this tendinitis and tenosynovitis picture is formed. The tenosynovitis may even be observed before the joint involvement. Tendinitis is the degeneration and inflammation of the tendons. As a result of the synovial fluid increase developing in the tendon sheaths, swelling of the sheaths and adhere to the tendons. Consequently the movement of the tendon in the sheath gets harder and this causes pain. Tenosynovitis is the inflammation of the tendon sheaths, in other words the parietal and visceral layers. As a result, this layers may adhere to each other or to the tendon and cause pain with joint motions. During the development of the tenosynovitis, fibrotic proliferation in the tendons, thickening in the synovial tissue and histopathological changes creating adhesion in the neighboring soft tissues are observed. Especially because of the evident reason of the inflammation, abnormality, deficiency and often pain develop in tendon functions. Clinically, pain and local sensitivity (which increases with tendon movement and the contraction of the related muscle), swelling, increase in local heat and redness, crepitation, decrease in ROM and muscle atrophy may develop. This picture which may develop are most often seen in the dorsal and volar surfaces of the wrist and volar surfaces of the fingers [8, 10, 11].

1. The dorsal (extensor) side of the wrist; swelling of the wrist is observed due to the dorsal wrist tenosynovitis (Figure 2). The pain is minimal; crepitation can be felt by palpation. It may involve one or several of the extensor tendons and be the first symptom of RA. In early stage spontaneous remission can be observed. In this group, the type called De Quervain stenozan tenosynovitis, which is seen in abductor pollisis longus (APL) and extensor pollisis brevis (EPB) tendons, is the most common. Most of the patients complain about the continuous pain which occur at the radial part of the wrist and the base of the thumb with the wrist motions and grabbing. In addition to the medical treatment of RA rest and if needed injections of steroids can be applied. If the tenosynovitis still continues despite a 4-6 months of conservative therapy, synovectomy as surgical treatment may be considered [8, 10].

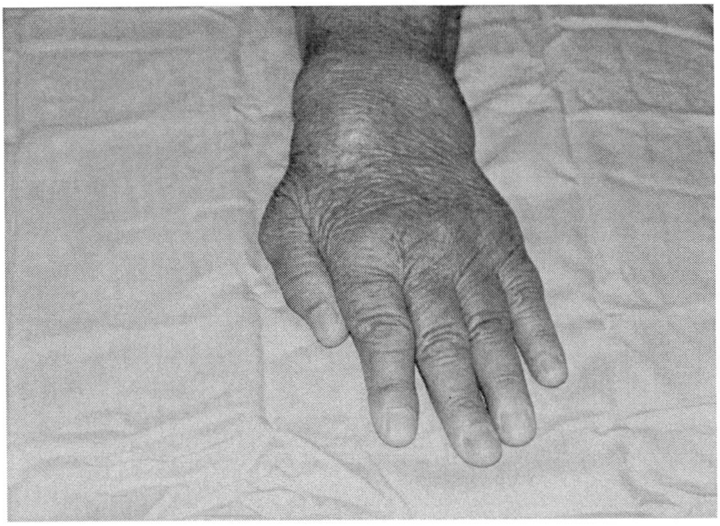

Figure 2. Synovitis and tenosynovitis on the radial side of the wrist

2. The volar (flexor) side of the wrist; in the volar side tenosynovitis of the wrist, the problem occurs inside the carpal tunnel, therefore the swelling is not as distinct as in the dorsal wrist tenosynovitis. Limitations in the passive and active ROM of the fingers may develop. This proliferative synovitis in the flexor tendon sheath may apply pressure to the median nerve and cause carpal tunnel syndrome [8, 10].
3. The volar surface of the fingers; pointed rheumatoid nodules are formed by the tenosynovitis of finger flexors in the tendons. Due to the existence of these nodules as well as the synovial hypertrophy, in the tendons which already pass through a narrow fibro-osseous canal, sticking occur (trigger finger). Intranodular injections are useful during the therapy. Tenosynovectomy and carpal tunnel loosening are applied for the patients who are not responding conservative treatment [8, 10].

2) Tendon Rupture

The main causes of tendon rupture in a rheumatoid hand are synovial invasion of the tendon and the chronic rubbing of the tendon over the especially eroded bones and a bony prominence. The rupture happens mostly at the termination site of the tendon and may be accompanied by fractures. Even though ruptures may occur in both dorsal and volar surfaces, extensor tendon ruptures are more common [10, 12].

The tendon ruptures in the dorsal side are observed most commonly in the distal side of the ulnar bone and the Lister's Tubercle [1]. The tubercles which develop alone on the extensor tendon can be seen in any finger but the little finger is effected most commonly. There, the tendon ruptures generally being rubbed up against the distal ulna. The rupture which develop in the little finger is frequently followed by the rupture in the ring finger and then the others [10]. This shows that the progress of the extensor tendon ruptures is from the ulnar to the radial direction and the rupture finally occurs at the second finger. These sequential ruptures in the extensor tendons occur rapidly. Another cause of the development of the rupture in the tendon is tenosynovitis. Tenosynovitis causes rupture by compressing the tendon and weakening the tendon by decreasing its blood supply [10]. The ruptures occur most frequently at extensor tendons, extensor pollicis longus (EPL), extensor digiti quinti and extensor digiti communis. EPL tendon rupture may not significantly affect the extension motion of the interphalangeal (IP) joint of the thumb by means of the intrinsic muscles. When the loss of significant level of deformity and functional restoration is observed in tendon ruptures surgical intervention may be needed. After the operation early passive mobilization is convenient as well as the splint support. In general, the results of the operations are better in single ruptures than multiple ruptures [1]. Clinically, extensor tendon ruptures may occur with an extension loss in metacarpophalangeal (MP) joint, but other reasons which cause the same picture such as ulnar tendon subluxation, MP joint dislocation and posterior interosseous nerve compression due to radiocapitellar synovitis should be excluded [1, 10]. It is difficult to distinguish tendon rupture from tendon paralysis. The most valid diagnostic maneuver is to evaluate MP joint extension while bringing the wrist to flexion (the tenodesis effect). Because of the lack of tendon integrity in a rupture, wrist flexion would not contribute the MP joint extension [10, 11].

Flexor pollisis longus (FPL), is the most frequently ruptured flexor tendon. Tendon typically gets ruptured while moving on the rough bulges of the scaphoid bone or trapezium. Patients can not actively move the thumb's IP joint. If there is a chronic stiffness or hyperextension at that joint, the diagnosis becomes more difficult. Similarly in the other fingers, the active flexion loss at the proximal interphalangeal (PIP) or distal interphalangeal (DIP) joints may respectively point to flexor digitorum superficialis (FDS) and flexor digitorum profundus (FDP) ruptures. Because the functional loss in FDS rupture alone is minimal it may not be repaired. If the DIP joint remains stable FDP ruptures may not be repaired, however in combined ruptures of FDP and FDS the functional loss is significant, therefore surgical intervention may be required [8, 10]. The early primary repair is important for all ruptures. For instance, if the ruptures developing in "no man's land", which is closely associated with superficial and deep flexor tendons (the limited palmar region between the distal palmar crease and PIP joints, where flexor tendons exist), are not repaired in the early period they may lead to ischemic necrosis. The most important problem after the repair of a tendon is the post-operative adhesions [10, 11]. In flexor tendon contrary to the extensor surface, the course of the rupture develops from the radial direction to the ulnar direction. After the rupture of FPL, the rupture occurs at the second finger tendon, then the third finger tendon and finally the little finger tendon [10]. Also, it has to be checked for a possible fracture [13].

3) Deformities and Subluxation

A. The Wrist Joint

At the wrist of the RA patients, distal radioulnar and radiocarpal joints get affected most; midcarpal joint gets affected relatively less [10, 11]. In early stage, synovial proliferation after the synovitis observed in these regions causes deformities at the wrist [10]. The changes observed in the rheumatoid wrist can be classified as clinical and radiological.

There are 4 clinical stages[14]:

1. Synovitis and osteopenic bone at the wrist.
2. Observation of radiologic erosion with limited wrist ROM and synovitis.
3. Observation of clinical and radiological significant subluxation, dislocation and/or joint destruction.
4. Ankylosis at the joint.

Larsen Classification is used radiologically [15].

Grade 0: Normal joint
Grade 1: Mild joint changes such as swelling of soft tissue, osteoporosis, and mild joint space narrowing
Grade 2: Observation of erosions besides the joint space narrowing.
Grade 3: Joint space narrowing and erosion at all joint
Grade 4: Serious destructive changes
Grade 5: Loss of the joint gap and bone deformities (mutilating changes).

Radiocarpal joint subluxation: Carpal bones can be subluxed from the distal radius in volar direction or ulnar direction or in both directions at the same time. The tendon of the extensor carpi ulnaris muscle slides to the volar surface of the joint and the extensor looses its function. This is called "caput ulnae syndrome" [10]. In caput ulnae syndrome, weakness in hand and wrist, limitation of the radioulnar joint rotation motion and pain during the motion, the relocation of styloid ridge of the ulna towards dorsal direction with painful crepitation, dorsal tenosynovitis and extensor tendon rupture are observed [16].

Radioulnar joint subluxation: Tendons do not hold on to carpal bones except for pisiformis and ligaments limit these bones. In RA these ligaments get weak and their stability disrupt. Weakening of the connection point of the ligament causes instability in the distal radioulnar joint. Distal part moves towards the dorsal and proximal part moves towards the volar causing deformity development [14].

Others: Followed by the synovitis observed in scafolunate joint and midcarpal joints, deformities develop. Ulnar translocation picture occurs as a consequence of the destruction of radiolunate and radiocarpal ligaments [10].

B. Metacarpophalangeal Joint

The MP joint, described as the key piece of the longitudinal and transfer arcs of hand, is the structure which is affected the most in RA patients and ulnar deviation as well as palmar subluxation deformity develop in these joints. Even though MPs are the preliminary joints involved, the ulnar deviation deformity is not usually observed in the early stage of the disease. The chances of observing this deformity increase for RA patients who have been diagnosed for 5 years or more [1, 10].

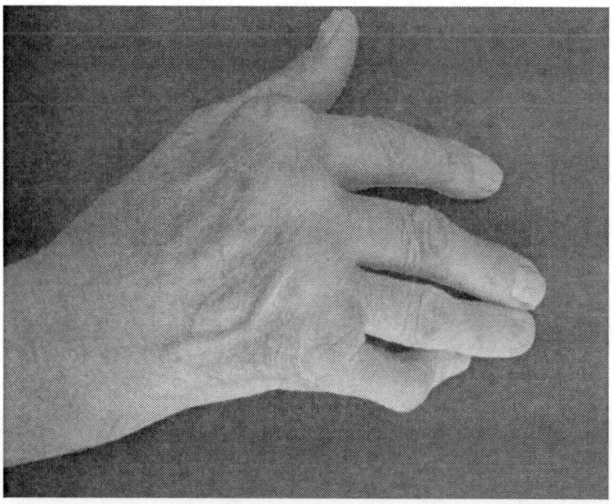

Figure 3. Ulnar deviation of metacarpophalangeal joints and radial deviation of the wrist and metacarpals

Ulnar deviation and palmar subluxation at the MP joints: MP joints allow the movement in both planes and they are more unstable than IF joints because of with their condylar structure. With the proliferation of synovium, joint capsule and ligamentous structures stretch and collateral ligaments loosen decreasing the joint stability. In addition to this, with the other factors affecting the MP joint such as wrist collapse, weak radiocarpal ligament and lateral pressure while the pinching activity of the thumb, characteristic ulnar deviation occurs [1,17] (Figure 3). The anatomical factors causing the development of the ulnar deviation deformity [11]:

- Radial lateral collateral ligaments being longer and thinner than ulnar collateral ligaments.
- Ulnar intrinsic muscles being bigger and advantageously placed compared to the radial intrinsic muscles.
- The heads of MP normally facing the ulnar direction.
- The flexor tendons applying a force on the fingers in the ulnar direction during the grasping and holding activities.
- The gravitational force helping the hand to go in the ulnar direction during the hand activities.

In addition to these, the synovitis developed at the hand of a RA patient may cause the wrist motion to go the radial direction by limiting the wrist motion towards the ulnar. Radial deviation of the metacarps and ulnar deviation of the fingers accompany that. This condition is known as the "zig-zag deformity" [17].

Also, the joint capsule being stretched because of the synovitis developed in the MKF joint is thought to cause "protective reflex spasm" in the interosseous and lumbrical muscles. The stress which occurs at the intrinsic muscles may cause "flexion contracture deformity", also known as "intrinsic plus position" [11, 17].

C. Finger Joint

In early acute stage of RA, the synovitis developed in PIF joint of the patients causes a painful and swollen joints especially in the mornings and also transforms the finger into a spindled shape. In next stages of the disease 'swan neck' and 'boutonniere' deformities occur (Figure 4).

Swan-neck deformity: Synovitis developed in any of the PIP, DIP and MP joints causes carpal collapse which bring along a muscle-tendon instability, and as a result 'swan neck deformity develops [10]. There are 4 types of swan neck deformity:

In type 1; the PIP joint may totally be flexed and the MP joint is minimally affected and its loss of function is minimal as well. First, due to the loss or the stress at the insertion point of extensor tendon, FDP tendon activity remains unopposed and the DIP joint flexes similarly to the mallet finger deformity. Relative shortness occurs in the lateral bands which move towards dorsal. Volar plate loosens at the PIP joint and transfers retinacular ligament thins down; PIP joint hyperextension occurs [11, 18].

In type 2; the pathology is in the MP joint. Due to the subluxation and ulnar deviation of MP joint, at the intrinsic muscles stress occurs; hyperextension at the PIP joint and flexion at the DIP joint develop. Bringing the MP joint to extension and to radial deviation at the physical examination limits the PIP joint flexion [11, 18].

In type 3; there is a fixed deformity. PIP joint flexion is limited in every position and hand functions worsen as the grasp weakens. Despite this functional loss, in X-ray significant joint destruction is not observed; because the flexion limitation develops depending mostly on the surrounding tissue. This condition should be considered at the treatment [11, 18].

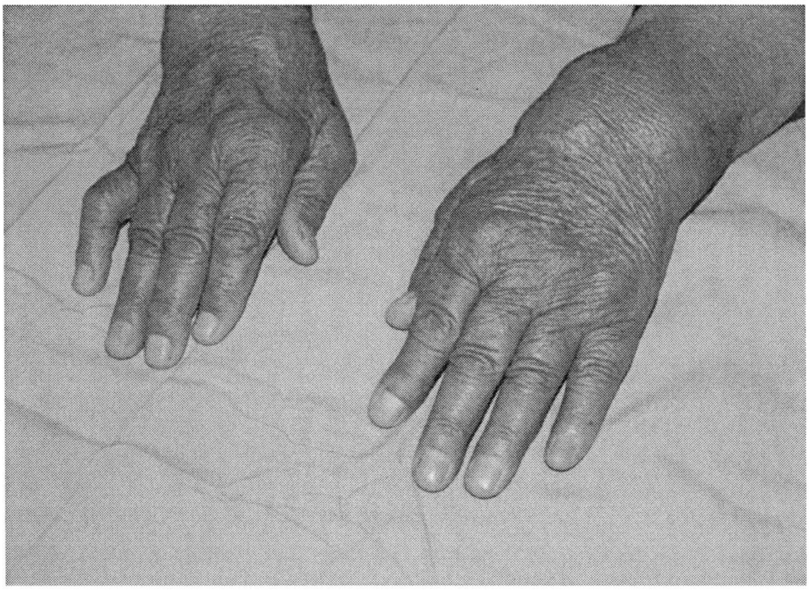

Figure 4. Swan-neck deformity on the left hand and boutonniere deformity on right hand in rheumatoid arthritis

In type 4; fixed deformity is accompanied by joint destruction [11, 18].

Boutonnière deformity: This deformity usually starts weakening and stressing the extensor mechanism by the synovial proliferation in the PIP joint [8, 11]. In the early stage or during a mild deformity, there is flexion in PIP joint (10-15° extension insufficiency) and minimal hyperextension in DIF joint [11]. In mid-level deformity; the flexion deformity in PIP joint is 30-40° and the hyperextension has already started in MP joint. In the mean time, in chronic stage or severe deformity cases; the hyperextension developed in MP accompanies the occurrence in order to compensate the flexion contracture in PIP joint. In severe deformities the active extension of the PIP joint can not be performed. Lateral bands move to volar and shortening happens in the oblique retinacular ligament which causes hyperextension of the DIP joint. This deformity is called 'boutonnière deformity', because lateral bands break away and allow to pass the joint between them. It is difficult to treat this deformity using conservative methods because of the rotation of lateral band causing the boutonnière deformity and the significant regression of the supporting fibrils [11, 19].

D. The Thumb

The deformities at the thumb due to RA occur in MP, IP and carpometacarpal (CMC) joints. There are 6 types of deformities due to RA in the thumb [1, 20, 21].

Type I: Boutonnière deformity that occurs PIP flexion, MP and DIP joint hyperextension is the more common type. The main problem is in the MP joint. CMC is not involved. The patient suffers especially pinching and grasping.

Type II: Flexion and adduction occur in the CMC joint, flexion occurs in the MP joint and hyperextension occurs in the IP joint. It is not very common. Z deformity occurs in case flexion develops in MP joint and extension develops only in PIP joint.

Type III: Swan neck deformity that occurs the subluxation, flexion and adduction of CMC joint, the hyperextension of MP joint and the flexion of IP joint is the second most common type of deformity.

Type IV: Flexion and adduction in CMC joint, hyperextension in MP joint and an unstable structure in the ulnar collateral ligaments are observed in this type. IP joint is not involved.

Type V: CMC is involved or it may be normal; MP volar plate is unstable. IP joint is not involved.

Type VI: There is a total resorption of bones in CMC, MP and IP joints (arthritis mutilans).

4) Entrapment Neuropathy

Carpal tunnel syndrome (CTS), is the most frequently entrapment neuropathy in RA. The tenosynovial proliferation in the flexor tendons increasing the pressure in the carpal tunnel causes compression on the median nerve; this leads to entrapment neuropathy [22]. The main point here is that it can be the first symptom of RA.

RA patient's hand functions are disrupted by the articular damage of the hand. This is compensated by adaptation mechanisms. If CTS also occurs, it becomes more difficult to continue this sensitive balance [6]. CTS prevalence of RA patients is noted to be between 23%-69 %. During its treatment splints, steroid injections, ultrasound, iontophoresis and low dose laser therapy can be used [23].

5) Nodule

The nodule development of RA patients is around 50 %. Most commonly it is observed along the tendons or at the joints, especially at the elbow joint. Nodules are composed of granulomatous and fibrous tissue. It reveals the severity of the disease. Nodules can be either painful or pain-free [10].

The Evaluation of the Hand Functions

Hand functions should be evaluated as global with regard to the individual's personal, professional and social needs. Although several methods are developed for this evaluation, most of them are not clinically practical [10]. Anamnesis and physical examination are crucial in hand evaluation. Besides this, there are measures and studies evaluating the functionality, damage and disability levels of the hand.

It is necessary to start the evaluation of rheumatoid hand by physical examination. Basically, during the physical examination the posture, edema, increase in local heat, ROM, skin color, muscle strenght, deformities, sensation and circulation of hand and wrist as well as the results of various special tests should be evaluated.

In physical examination, the inspection should start by looking for deformity, edema and possible color change in the hand.

It is argued that most of the deformities develop in early stage and that they may be clinically useful in determining the severity of the disease. For this reason the evaluation of hand deformities should not be neglected in RA patients [24]. The palpation of hand and wrist is a helpful examination method to determine either the deformities are corrected or not, subluxated or dislocated [10].

In order to determine the edema which has an important role in hand functions precisely beside the inspection, hand volumeters may be used [25]. Considering the significant limitation of active ROM and the hand functions caused by the inflammatory symptoms, the early detection of the edema would provide an early intervention with the inflammation.

In RA, due to disrupted power balance around the joint, contractures and muscle shortening occur. For this reason RA patients should be active and passive ROM examination. In the hand-wrist ROM; flexion (80-90°), extension (60-70°), ulnar deviation (30-40°), radial deviation (15-20°), pronation and supination (80-90°) are evaluated. In the thumb ROM; at the CMC joint flexion- extension (40-50°) and adduction-abduction (0- 40-70 °); at the MKF joint flexion (50-70°) and extension (10-30°); at the IP joint flexion (50-90°) and extension (20-35°) are evaluated. The thumb touches all the fingers during the opposition. In the fingers besides thumb, MP joints allow 90° flexion, 30° extension and 35° radial and ulnar motions. PIP joints allow 100-120° flexion. DIP joint allows 50-80° flexion and 5-10° extension. In abduction fingers diverge approximately 20° with equal distance. In a normal hand, when the wrist is in flexion, the fingers and the thumb are in extension; when the wrist is in extension, fingers are in flexion (tenodesis effect) [10, 11].

Hand deformities with the other deficits, such as reduced grasping force and the pain, are very effective on the hand functions and the activities of daily life [24, 26]. Besides, there would be muscle weakness due to the factors such as power imbalance around the joints and entrapment neuropathy; therefore muscle strength test is required for these patients. Manuel muscle test may be misleading in early stage, so the results obtained by a hand dynamometer would be more accurate for the evaluation of the muscle strength [27]. The basic measures of muscle strength in the hand are; grip (three fingers or three points, lateral or key and with finger tips) and grasp (cylindrical, spherical and hook) strenghts. Most of the RA patients have less muscle strength compared with healthy individuals, consequently their daily activities are much more limited [26, 28]. There is a high correlation between the grasping strength and difficulty in activities of daily life [28, 29]. Determining the weaknesses of the hand-wrist muscles may give us an idea about the condition of the hand functions and may help us to decide about the use of the supportive device [28]. The flexion loss at the joint has a more important role in hand functionality than the extension. One of the most effective measurements to evaluate the joint flexion is specific grasping. The flexion loss of the 2nd and 3rd MP joints usually causes a small functional loss, while a little flexion loss in the 4th and 5th MP joints leads to significant functional loss. The mild flexion loss of PIP joint is tolerated well [11, 28]. Ulnar deviation does not cause a significant loss in hand functions in early stage, but eventually it becomes a determinant factor over the hand functioning. Swan neck deformity has a more effective role over hand functions than the boutonnière deformity [24]. Extension loss does not develop often at the joint; in case it develops it restrains the grasping of big objects. But by the time, extension loss causes flexion deformity, therefore functional loss [10]. These deformities affect on the general functions beside the hands. In ten years, one or more deformities develop in more than half of the patients. The development of deformity gives us an idea about the severity of the disease. However, there are not clear results about how often been seen in which deformities [24].

In sensory examination, light touch, pressure, proprioception, two points discrimination test and pick-up test are evaluated. In order to get objective results in this examination, the use of portable devices would be convenient [30].

There are measurements and examinations which evaluate the pathological development process in the rheumatoid hand in a functional level, observing its radiological effect on the wrist and hand joints [31]. Let us give some examples of most commonly used methods. One of the methods measuring the influence of hand functions on the daily life is The Health Assessment Questionnaire (HAQ) [32]. This measure is evaluated the degree of disability of the patients. However, Duruoz Hand Scale, which is a easy to use, a high performance measure and developed specifically for the rheumatoid hand, may be used to evaluate the insufficiency of the hand functions [33]. The Rheumatoid Arthritis Articular Damage (RAAD) score is commonly used to evaluate the articular damage and deformities in RA [34]. For the structural joint damages in the radiographies Modified Sharp Score is utilized. There are some imaging methods to determine the level of the damage of the hand in early stages of RA such as magnetic resonance imaging (MRI), three dimensional computer tomography and ultrasonography. For instance, MRI determines the hypertrophy in synovium within the four months after the synovitis starts [12, 35].

Rehabilitation of the Rheumatoid Hand

The main purposes of the rehabilitation are to control the pain and inflammation, to provide and maintain the joint mobilization, to prevent the deformities and to help the daily activities by increasing the functional capacity. Also, the treatment should be personalized for the patient and the existing or potential deformities should be structured considering the stage of the disease and the daily needs. During the treatment it is important for the patients to be informed about the disease and treatment options [10].

The most important point while planning the treatment is the stage of the disease; because the treatment options are decided according to these stages [10].

Stage I: acute stage where the inflammation exists. There is swelling, heat, pain and redness at the joints.

Stage II: sub-acute stage where the synovial proliferation is observed. Due to the proliferation, the mobility decreases and the pain decreases as well.

Stage III: chronic stage where the destruction starts. Deformities of soft tissue and joint are observed.

Stage IV: there are serious deformities, subluxation and fusion at hand and wrist.

The role of the physiotherapy for the rheumatologic patients is still argued. There are many physical therapy methods such as hot-cold applications, electrical currents like transcutaneous electrical nerve stimulation (TENS), laser, hydrotherapy and exercise therapy. Paraffin and sulfide baths are efficient and reliable especially for RA patients. The common effects of these methods are extension of the collagens, decrease of the joint involvement, muscle spasm relief and increase of the blood circulation. Especially paraffin is very beneficial for the RA hand. Exercise applied after the use of paraffin increase its positive effect. The same way, the hot-cold packs applications have a very positive effect on the inflammation, and grasping functions and decrease the pain and the swelling. These applications actually aim to increase the comfort and exercise performance of the patient [36]. During the acute stage, cold applications; during the chronic stage hot applications should be chosen [11]. In RA patients TENS is preferred because of its analgesic effect [37]. With its non-thermal effects besides its thermal effects, the ultrasound treatment is one of the useful physical therapy methods in RA. Applied as phonophorosis, it is observed to be more successful in suppression of inflammation in the RA hand [38]. However, besides all these physical treatment modalities, exercise programs which are proven to be beneficial in rheumatoid hand should be applied [36].

The functional use of hand without pain for RA patients during activities of daily life is important. Exercise has an important role to provide and protect that. With the application of the exercise program; the joint mobility and functional capacity is protected, the pain and involvement of the joint decrease, advanced deformities are prevented. Hammond and Freeman [39] did one year follow up study that demonstrated the positive effects of joint protection program on the pain, disease condition and functional capacity. In their study Buljina et al. [36] applied physical treatment (thermal bath, faradic bath, therapeutic hot or cold bath depending on the condition of inflammation and exercise therapy) to 50 of the 100 patients; then evaluated the other 50 as the control group. At the end of three weeks, they observed significant progress of ROM, Ritchie hand articular index, pain scale, grasping and pinching strength in the physical treatment group compared with the control group. In a study they made to evaluate the rheumatoid hand treatment, O'Brien et al. [2] divided 67 patients into three groups. They only educated one of the groups, applied stretching exercise program and the education to the second group and finally strengthening and mobilization home exercise program in addition to the education to the last group. At the end of 6 months the Arthritis Impact Measurement Scale-II (AIMS II) evaluations of the group subjected to strengthening and mobilization exercises showed a significant progress compared with the other two. With this study and other similar ones the exercise programs given to RA patients are determined. During the acute period with the inflammation, in order to protect the ROM active- assistive exercises are applied up to the pain limit, once or twice a day. Even in this period rest is not commonly suggested. After the decrease of the inflammation the exercise program is rearranged in order to increase the active ROM and protect the muscle strength. The purpose of the exercises done during the chronic period is to increase the functional use of hand. Hand activities composed of active joint movements may be applied. If intense pain occurs during the exercise, and continues after an hour of the exercise with the inflammation at the joint, it can be concluded that the program is not convenient. In that case the frequency and intensity of the exercise should be decreased [2, 10]. While giving RA patients an exercise program for hand and wrist, passive exercises should be avoided as much as possible or they should be applied very carefully. If intensive force is applied on a joint and the pain limit is exceeded, the joint and neighboring tissues which are already biomechanically disrupted would get damaged more. The fact that the main purpose of the exercise programs is to gain pain-free hand functions back should always be remembered. Therefore, resistant and compulsive exercises should not be applied in order to increase the grasping strength of the advanced rheumatoid hand deformity. Otherwise due to the deformity, the hand functions get negatively affected. When the joint motions are accompanied by pain, isometric exercises should be preferred to isotonic exercises. That way, the muscle strength may be protected and increased without pain. To prevent the contractures or to increase the ROM after the contracture develops in RA hand stretching exercises are applied. Stretching exercise should be applied as active stretching. The stretching exceeding the pain limit should be avoided. When the result of active stretching is unsatisfying techniques as serial casting and splinting may be used. To perform the exercise program more efficiently, hot or cold applications may be helpful. Because of the contradictory information about the intensity of the exercise programs, it is hard to have a clear opinion [40-43]. The results of the studies about this issue are not satisfactory [28].

Occupational therapy programs given in addition to the exercise programs especially at the early stage of RA affect the hand functions positively. The activities of daily life and work environment are modified with these programs. The patients are informed about the assistive devices, joint protection techniques and methods to decrease the energy consumption. The studies show that the occupational therapy has a positive effect on the activities of daily life of RA patients and increases the functional capacity [44-46].

In RA; ring splints, ulnar deviation splints, postoperative dynamic splints, rest splints for CTS and pain-inflammation control and thumb splints which decrease the CMK joint stress may be used and contribute the rehabilitation. For a patient in stage 1, use of a rest splint at night and part-time in the day would be convenient in order to prevent potential deformities and decrease the pain and inflammation. In stage 2; the night use of the rest splint is recommended in order to prevent deformity development. In stage 3; splints that can prevent the progress of an advanced deformity and protect against the potential deformities are preferred. In stage 4; with the use of finger and wrist splints against advanced deformities the joint may be kept stable during the daily activities [10] (Table 1). However, there is not precise knowledge about the use of many splints in RA yet. The information about the effects of the working splints of wrist on the functionality and the pain are not sufficient. It is also argued that some splints decrease the grasping strength and hand ability. Some studies showed that the rest splints and others do not have any effect on the ROM and pain, therefore they are not preferred by the patients [47]. Some other studies stated that the use of the ring splint increases the patient's hand ability and is particularly helpful in mobile swan neck deformity [48, 49]. It is noted that the splint is not protective in fast progressing cases, yet it reduces the pain. The uses of the splints which provide positioning at night are useful in terms of functions and pain [50]. Besides its effects on the pain and deformity, splints have other benefits such as protecting the hand against excessive internal and external traumatic forces, helping to perform daily activities more comfortably, preventing the progress of the muscle atrophy, reducing the formation of contractures and supporting the exercises on the weakened muscles. With the use of the assistive devices and the modifications within the house, the daily life activities of the patients would get easier [10].

The treatment should be planned according to the stage of the disease. The purpose in stage 1 is to reduce the pain and the inflammation. For this reason, when the hand and wrist of a RA patient is determined to be in active period, in order to control the inflammation and pain at the joint and the surrounding structures the hand is immobilized. Therefore, the splints should be used in convenient positions close to the functional position to prevent the development of deformities, to help the inflamed structures to rest and to support them [10]. However, to leave the patient immobilized for a long time would not be a right approach. Therefore, the pain and inflammation should be controlled as soon as possible by using physical treatment methods such as, application of cold, TENS, laser, suitable exercise program and local injections of steroids [10, 51]. Even during acute period, the muscle strength should be protected by static isometric exercises and the splints should be taken of 3-

4 times a day in order to do ROM exercises [10]. The goal in the stage 2 is to provide the continuance of active ROM, to avoid the positions which may cause deformity and to reduce joint traumas. Therefore, in this stage active ROM exercises and physical treatment methods should be applied. In chronic stage, the goal is to prevent the progress of existing deformities, to protect existing functions and to increase the functionality. For this reason, in addition to the ROM exercise endurance and strength exercises and other methods of physical therapy should be applied. In addition to this, modification of the working methods, balancing the energy consumption, use of assistive devices and patient education about all these should be part of the rehabilitation [8, 10].

Table 1. The Principles Of Treatment According To Stages Of Rheumatoid Arthritis

Stage I	The aim is to reduce the pain and the inflammation.
	The hand is immobilized.
	Resting splint is used.
	Physical therapy modalities are used.
	Static isometric exercises are applied
Stage II	The aim is to provide the continuance of active ROM, to avoid the deformity and to reduce joint traumas
	Night splint is used.
	Physical therapy modalities are used.
	Static isometric and active ROM exercises are applied
Stage III	The aim is to prevent the progress of the deformity and to avoid the deformity
	Night and funcitonal day splints are used.
	Physical therapy modalities are used.
	Static isometric, strength and active ROM exercises are applied
Stage IV	The aim is to prevent the progress of the deformity, to protect existing functions and to increase the functionality
	Different type splints are used.
	Physical therapy modalities are used.
	Static isometric, strength, endurance and active ROM exercises are applied

Patients should be guided for an operation at the right time. Intensive pain, increase of disability, progress of joint damages and significant insufficiency of the hand functions effecting daily life activities are surgical indications. Tenosynovectomies, repairs of extensor and flexor tendon ruptures, tendon transfers, distal ulna excisions, reconstruction of the distal radioulnar joint complex, hand-wrist fusion, deregulation of intrinsic muscles and joint aortoplasty are the possible surgical processes [52, 53].

Conclusion

In conclusion; RA is a chronic disease which is characterized by synovial inflammation. Hand and wrist are frequently involved and tendinitis, tenosynovitis, tendon ruptures, deformity, entrapment neuropathy and nodules occur. These developing problems disrupt the hand balance; therefore they cause weakness, pain and functional loss at the hand. Therefore the hand-wrist examination is crucial for RA patients. The goal in the treatment is to prevent the deterioration of deformity and to conserve the hand functionality by controlling the pain and inflammation. Medical treatment, physical therapy modalities, exercise programs, occupational therapy, splints and surgical applications when required are the main treatment applications.

References

[1] Wang, AA; Weiland, AJ. *Surgery of arthritic deformities of the hand. In:Koopman WJ editor. Arthritis and Allied Conditions.* 14th edition. Philadelphia: Lippincott Williams&Wilkins, 2001, 989-1002.

[2] O'Brien, AV; Jones, P; Mullis, R; Mulherin, D; Dziedzic, K. Conservative hand therapy treatments in rheumatoid arthritis. *Rheumatology,* 2006, 45, 577–83.

[3] Bodur, H; Yilmaz, O; Keskin, D. Hand disability and related variables in patients with rheumatoid arthritis. *Rheumatol Int,* 2006, 26, 541-544.

[4] Towheed, TE; Anastassiades, TP. Rheumatoid hand practical approach to assessment and management. *Can Fam Physician,* 1994, 40, 1303-1309.

[5] Dellhag, B; Bjelle, A. A five-year followup of hand function and activities of daily living in rheumatoid arthritis. *Arthritis Care Res,* 1999, 2, 33–41.

[6] Barnes, CG; Currey, HL. Carpal tunnel syndrome in rheumatoid arthritis a clinical and electrodiagnostic survey. *Ann Rheum Dis,* 1967, 26, 226-233.

[7] Apfelberg, DB; Maser, MR; Lash, H; Kaye, RL; Britton, MC; Bobrove, A. Rheumatoid hand deformities: Patophysiology and treatment. *West J Med,* 1978, 129, 267-272.

[8] Gordon, DA; Hastings, DE. Clinical features of rheumatoid arthritis. In: MC Hochberg, AJ Silman, JS Smolen, ME Weinblatt, MH Weisman editors. *Rheumatology.* Fourth Edition. Elsevier; 2008, 770-779.

[9] Firestein, GS. Pathogenesis of rheumatoid arthritis: how early is early? *Arthritis Res Ther,* 2005, 7, 157-159.

[10] Mackin, EJ; Callahan, AD; Osterman, AL; Skirven, TM; Schneider, LH; Hunter, JM. *Hunter, Mackin & Callahan's Rehabilitation of the Hand and Upper Extremity.* 5th Edition. St.Louis, Mo: Mosby; 2002.

[11] Cailliet, Rene. *Hand Pain and Impairment.* 3th Edition. Philadelphia: F A: Davis Co; 1982

[12] Ishikawa, H; Abe, A; Murasawa, A; Nakazono, K; Horizono, H; Ishii, K; Seki, E. Rheumatoid wrist deformity and risk of extensor tendon rupture evaluated by 3DCT imaging. *Skeletal Radiol,* 2010, 7.

[13] Schneider, AB. Rehabilitation of the Wrist, Hand and Finger. In: Prentice WE, Voigth ML, editors. *Techniques in Musculoskeletal Rehabilitation.* NY: McGraw-Hill Medical Publishing Division; 2001, 499-505.
[14] Taleisnik, J. *The Wrist.* New York: Churchill Livingstone; 1985.
[15] Larsen, A; Dale, K; Eek, M. Radiographic evaluation of rheumatoid arthritis by Standard reference films. *Acta Radiol Diagn*, 1977, 18, 481-91.
[16] Backdahl, M. The caput ulnae syndrome in rheumatoid arthritis: a study of the morphology, abnormal anatomy, and clinical picture. *Acta Rheumatol Scand,* 1963, 5, 1-75.
[17] Bielefeld, T; Neumann, DA. The unstable metacarpophalangeal joint in rheumatoid arthritis: anatomy, pathomechanics, and physical rehabilitation considerations.. *J Orthop Sports Phys Ther*, 2005, 35, 502-520.
[18] Nalebuff, EA. The rheumatoid swan-neck deformity. *Hand Clin*, 1989, 5, 203-214.
[19] Ferlic, DC. Boutonniere deformities in rheumatoid arthritis. *Hand Clin*, 1989, 5, 215-222.
[20] Nalebuff, EA. The rheumatoid thumb. *Clin Rheum Dis*, 1984, 10, 589-607.
[21] Stein, AB; Terrono, AL. The rheumatoid thumb. *Hand Clin* 1996, 12, 541-550.
[22] Shinoda, J; Hashizume, H; McCown, C; Senda, M; Nishida, K; Doi, T; Inoue, H. Carpal tunnel syndrome grading system in rheumatoid arthritis. *J Orthop Sci*, 2002, 7, 188-193.
[23] Ekim, A; Armagan, O; Tascioglu, F; Oner, C; Colak, M. Effect of low level laser therapy in rheumatoid arthritis patient with carpal tunnel syndrome. *Swiss Med Wkly*, 2007, 137, 347-352.
[24] Johnsson, PM; Eberhardt, K. Hand deformities are important signs of disease severity in patients with early rheumatoid arthritis. *Rheumatology,* 2009, 48, 1398-1401.
[25] Waylett-Rendall, J; Seibly, DS. A study of the accuracy of a commercially available volumeter. *Work,* 2007, 22, 107-110.
[26] Dellhag, B; Burckhardt, CS. Predictors of hand function in patients with rheumatoid arthritis. *Arthritis Care Res,* 1995, 8, 16-20.
[27] Cooper, H; Dodds, WN; Adams, ID; DeDombal, FT; Steele, VA.. Use and misuse of the tape measure as a means of assessing muscle strength and power. *Rheumatol Rehabil*, 1981, 20, 211-218.
[28] Rønningen, A; Kjeken, I.Effect of an intensive hand exercise programme in patients with rheumatoid arthritis. *Scand J Occup Ther*, 2008, 15, 173-183.
[29] Thyberg; I; Hass, UA; Nordenskiold, U; Gerdle, B; Skogh, T. Activity limitation in rheumatoid arthritis correlates with reduced grip force regardless of sex: The Swedish TIRA Project. *Arthritis Rheum*, 2005, 53, 886-896.
[30] Horch, K; Hardy, M; Jimenez, S; Jabaley, M. An automated tactile tester for evaluation of cutaneous sensibility. *J Hand Surg* 1992, 17, 829-837.
[31] Helliwel, P; Howe, A; Wright, V. Functional assessment of the hand: reproducibility, acceptability and utility of a new system for measuring strength. *Ann Rheum Dis,* 1987, 46, 203-208.
[32] Sokka, T; Kautiainen, H; Hannonen, P; Pincus T. Changes in Health Assessment Questionnaire disability scores over five years in patients with rheumatoid arthritis compared with the general population. *Arthritis Rheum,* 2006, 54, 3113-3118.

[33] Duruöz, MT; Poiraudeau, S; Fermenian, J; Menkes, CJ; Amor, B; Dougados, M; Revel, M. Development and validation of a rheumatoid hand functional disability scale that assesses functional handicap. J Rheumatol, 1996, 23, 1167-1172.

[34] Hulsmans, HM; Jacobs, JW;Van der Heijde, DM; Van Albada-Kuipers, GA; Schenk, Y; Bijlsman, JM. The course of radıologıc damage durıng the first six years of rheumatoid arthritis. *Arthritis Rheum*, 2000, 43, 1927-1940.

[35] Lee, DM; Weinblatt, ME. Rheumatoid arthritis. *Lancet,* 2001, 358, 903-911.

[36] Buljina, AI; Taljanovic, MS; Avdic, DM; Hunter, TB. Physical and Exercise Therapy for Treatment of the Rheumatoid Hand. *Arthritis Rheum*, 2001, 45, 392-397.

[37] Brosseau, L; Judd, MG; Marchand, S; Robinson, VA; Tugwell, P; Wells, G; Yonge K. Transcutaneous electrical nerve stimulation (TENS) for the treatment of rheumatoid arthritis in the hand. *Cochrane Database Syst Rev,* 2003, CD004377

[38] Hsieh, YL. Effects of ultrasound and diclofenac phonophoresis on inflammatory pain relief: suppression of inducible nitric oxide synthase in arthritic rats. *Phys Ther*, 2006, 86, 39-49.

[39] Hammond, A; Freeman, K. One-year outcomes of a randomized controlled trial of an educational-behavioural joint protection programme for people with rheumatoid arthritis. *Rheumatology,* 2001, 40, 1044-1051.

[40] De Jong, Z; Vliet Vlieland, TP. Safety of exercise in patients with rheumatoid arthritis. *Curr Opin Rheumatol*, 2005, 17, 177-182.

[41] De Jong, Z; Munneke, M; Zwinderman, AH; Kroon, HM; Ronday, KH; Lems, WF; Dijkmans, BA; Breedveld, FC; Vliet Vlieland, TP; Hazes, JM; Huizinga, TW. Long term high intensity exercise and damage of small joints in rheumatoid arthritis. *Ann Rheum Dis,* 2004, 63: 1399-1405.

[42] Van den Ende, CH; Vliet Vlieland, TP; Munneke, M; Hazes, JM. Dynamic exercise therapy in rheumatoid arthritis: A systematic review. *Br J Rheumatol*, 1998, 37, 677-687.

[43] Brorsson, S; Hilliges, M; Sollerman, C; Nilsdotter, A A six-week hand exercise programme improves strength and hand function in patients with rheumatoid arthritis. *J Rehabil Med*, 2009, 41, 338-342.

[44] Clark, BM. Rheumatology: 9. Physical and occupational therapy in the management of arthritis. *CMAJ,* 2000, 163, 999-1005.

[45] Helewa, A; Goldsmith, CH; Lee, P; Bombardier, C; Hanes, B; Smythe, HA; Tugwell, P. Effects of occupational therapy home service on patients with rheumatoid arthritis. *Lancet* 1991, 337:1453-6.

[46] Rapoliene, J; Krisciunas, A. The effectiveness of occupational therapy in restoring the functional state of hands in rheumatoid arthritis patients. *Medicana (Kaunas)* 2006, 42, 823-288.

[47] Egan, M; Brosseau, L; Farmer, M; Ouimet, MA; Ress, S; Tugwell, P; Wells, GA. *Splints and Orthosis for treating rheumatoid arthritis*. The Cochrane Library, 2001, Issue 1.

[48] Ziljstra,TR; Heinjnsdijk-Rouwenhorst, L; Raske, JJ. Silver ring splints improve dexterity in patients with rheumatoid arthritis. Arthritis Rheum, 2004, 51, 947-951.

[49] van der Giesen, FJ; van Lankveld, WJ; Kremers-Selten, C; Peeters, AJ; Stern, EB; Le Cessie, S; Nelissen, RG; Vliet Vlieland, TP. Effectiveness of two finger splints for

swan neck deformity in patients with rheumatoid arthritis: a andomized, crossover trial. *Arthritis Rheum,* 2009, 15: 1025-1031.

[50] Silva, AC; Jones, A; Silva, PG; Natour, J. Effectiveness of a night-time hand positioning splint in rheumatoid arthritis: a randomized controlled trial. *J Rehabil Med,* 2008, 40, 749-754.

[51] Meireles, SM; Jones, A; Jennings, F; Suda, AL; Parizotto, NA; Natour, J. Assessment of the effectiveness of low-level laser therapy on the hands of patients with rheumatoid arthritis: a randomized double-blind controlled trial. *Clin Rheumatol*, 2010, 16.

[52] Chung, KC; Kotsis, AV; Kim, HM; Burke, FD; Wilgis, EFS. Reasons why rheumatoid arthritis patients seek surgical treatment for hand deformities. *J Hand Surg Am*, 2006, 31, 289-294.

[53] Jain, A; Witbreuk, M; Ball, C; Nanchahal, J. Influence of steroids and methotrexate on wound complications after elective rheumatoid hand and wirst surgery. *J Hand Surg*, 2002, 27, 449-455.

In: Rheumatoid Arthritis: Prevalence, Risk…
Editor: Michael H. Madsen
ISBN: 978-1-61761-931-1

Chapter 4

Relevance of Genetic Risk Factors in Rheumatoid Arthritis

Jezabel Varadé, Emilio Gómez de la Concha and Elena Urcelay
Departament of Clinical Immunology, Hospital Clínico San Carlos, Madrid, Spain

Abstract

Rheumatoid arthritis (RA) is an autoimmune disease that affects approximately 1% of the population worldwide. RA etiology is complex, with both genetic and environmental factors influencing predisposition. Twin and family studies suggest that around 60% of heritability is due to genetic factors, being the *HLA-DRB1 locus* in he major histocompatibility complex (MHC) the main contributor [1]. The shared epitope (SE) hypothesis pointed to a short amino acid sequence common to all *HLA-DRB1* alleles as the primary susceptibility factor associated with RA [2]. This region has been consistently associated with RA across all populations. However, it is unclear whether the MHC *locus* predisposes to RA *per se* or owing to the development of anti-citrullinated peptide antibodies, which in turn would predispose to RA [3].

Different approaches have been used in the past to identify the genes associated with RA outside of the MHC. One effective approach to discover risk alleles in RA has been the candidate gene approach. This kind of studies led to the description of the tyrosine-phospatase gene *PTPN22* as a susceptibility factor for RA [4].

The identification of the *STAT4* polymorphism rs7574865 as a susceptibility factor for RA is an example of a combined strategy between linkage and case-control studies. Initially, Remmers *et al.* [5] selected candidate genes from a linkage region of 52 Mb on chromosome 2q, previously defined by Amos *et al* [6]. They performed the corresponding fine mapping, and the top associated marker, rs7574865, maped to the *STAT4* gene.

During the past 3 years, SNP genotyping technologies of high throughput have allowed investigators to efficiently screen common variation across the human genome [7, 8], Genome–wide association studies (GWAS) combined this technology with large case-control collections to identify associated alleles. Several associations at *TRAF1-C5,*

6q23, *TNFAIP3* or *REL loci* have been independently described by this kind of analysis [9-12].

Although much of the recent excitement in the field has resulted from the utilization of GWAS to search for genes outside the MHC, it is important to remember some things. Firstly, the single most important contribution to genetic risk for RA clearly resides within the MHC. Secondly, validated non-MHC RA risk alleles only explain 5% of the genetic weight of disease, and finally, GWAS had been performed at European ancestry cohorts so it will be of particular interest to conduct these GWAS in collections of non-European ancestry [3, 13].

In summary, approximately half of the genetic susceptibility to RA remains to be explained at present [3, 13].

Introduction

Rheumatoid arthritis (RA) is a chronic inflammatory joint disease, characterized by multiple diarthroididal joints leading to pain, deformities and a reduced quality of life. The aetiology of RA has not been fully established, but epidemiologic data clearly reflects a complex genetic component and presumably variable contributions by environmental factors. Separately, each genetic factor makes only a modest contribution to the overall genetic risk of developing a given complex disease.

We describe here the most important genetic factors that have been identified as influencing the occurrence of the disease. Some of these factors have also been studied as possibly associated with the course and severity of RA.

Epidemiology

The prevalence of RA in the general population ranges from 0.2 to 1%. The incidence of RA is different across populations, a considerable variation of the disease frequency has been reported among different populations. Some ethnic and racial groups like Pima Indians [14], have an increased occurrence of the disease with a prevalence rate of more than 2%, by contrast a very low prevalence of less than 0.3% has been reported in Asian populations [15]. Studies from South European countries also suggest a relative lower occurrence of RA when compared with North European and North American countries [15]. The prevalence of the disease appears to be lower in developing countries like some areas of rural Africa [16].

It has been suggested that RA in Southern Europe has a particular genetic, epidemiological and clinical profile [17].

RA is far more common in women than in men, the female-to-male ratio being 3:1. However, the mechanism to explain how gender influences the susceptibility to RA remains unclear. Differences in sex hormones may be involved [18].

Genetic Risk Factors

Several steps are involved in the investigation of complex disease aetiology. First, enough evidence must be accumulated to suggest a role for genetic factors in the disease. Familial aggregation constitutes indirect support for an influence of genetic factors.

First-Degree Relatives

Family studies seek to suggest the existence of an inherited component in the development of a specific disease by showing that cases cluster within families. An increased rate of the disease among first-degree relatives of affected individuals (parents, siblings and children) compared to the general population is taken as evidence of an inherited component. A useful measure is the relative risk λ, defined as the ratio of the rate of disease in first-degree relatives of a patient compared to the rate in general population [19].

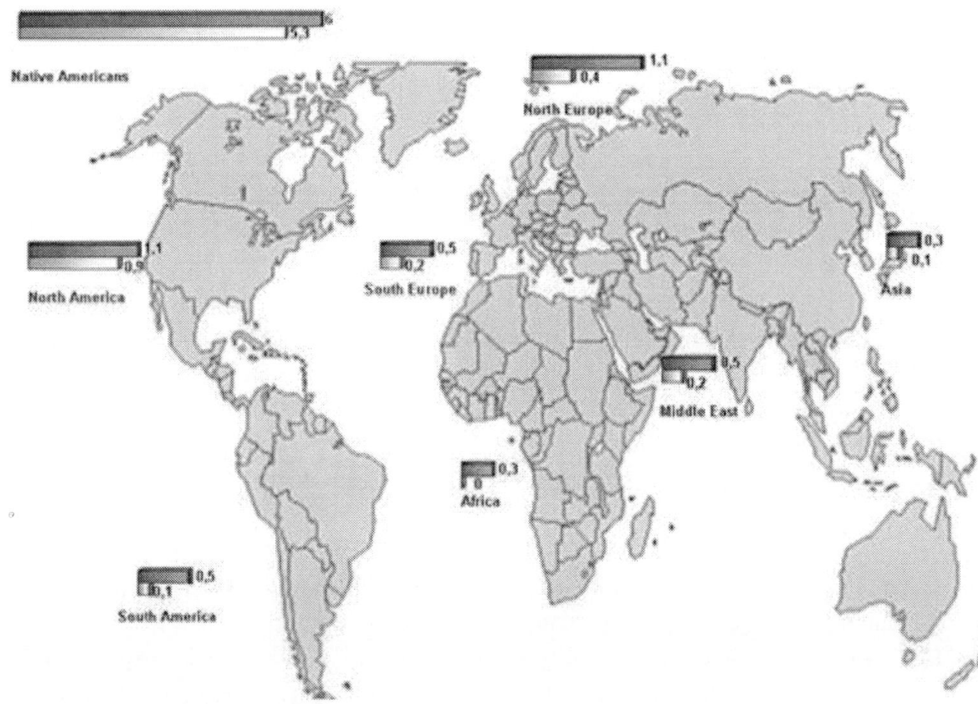

Figure 1. Prevalence of RA worldwide (cases per 100 inhabitants) [15]

The prevalence of RA among first-degree relatives of patients ranges from 2 to 12% [20]. In RA λs ("S" from "sibling"), is estimated at 3 to 15 [21, 22].

Twin Studies

Twin studies provide valuable information on the genetic component of multifactorial diseases. They compare the concordance rate (proportion of twin pairs in which both twins are affected) between monozygotic and dizygotic pairs.

Twin studies have been performed to estimate the genetic contribution to RA development. An increased rate of disease among monozygotic twins compared with dizygotic twins offers evidence in support of inherited factors predisposing to disease risk; the analysis of twin studies suggests that RA is approximately 65% heritable [1]. Given that the concordance between monozygotic twins is far from 100%, the influence of environmental factors in RA predisposition seems plausible.

The Major Histocompatibility Complex (MHC)

To date, the main genetic contributor to RA susceptibility remains the *HLA-DRB1 locus* in the Major Histocompatibility Complex (MHC) region. The MHC region, located at 6p21, is one of the most studied regions in the human genome due to its association with several autoimmune diseases. In 1978 Stastny et al [23]. described the first association between the HLA-Dw4 serotype and RA risk. The development of new serological and molecular techniques allowed the ascertainment of the *HLA-DRB1*0401* allele (corresponding to the HLA-Dw4 serotype from Stastny *et al.* description) in Caucasians.

In the 1980s, Gregersen et al [2], proposed the "shared epitope" (SE) hypothesis. They anticipated that different DRβ1 molecules share the same DNA sequence; and all these molecules might bind the same susceptibility epitope. As a result of this antigenic presentation, RA patients would develop autoreactive T-cells. Nowadays, the following *HLA-DRB1* alleles: *DRB1*0101, *0102, *0401, *0404, *0405, *0408*, **1001* and **1402* are accepted to be associated with RA risk. All of them share a conserved nucleotide sequence that codifies to an aminoacid sequence located in the third hypervariable region from DRβ1 molecule. In this model, the motifs QKRAA and RRRAA predispose to RA by influencing antigenic peptide presentation [2]. These residues are critical determinants of the so-called p4 peptide-binding pocket of the DRβ1 molecule. Due to the positively charged K/R at position 71, this pocket has a high affinity for negatively charged or uncharged polar residues[24]. It is supposed that the epitopes presented by these molecules are citrullinated peptides.

Citrulline is a post-translational modification of arginine. In the presence of high calcium concentration the enzyme peptidyl arginine deiminase (*PAD*), which is present in granulocytes and monocytes, converts the positively charged iminogroup of arginine to the uncharged carbonyl group of citrulline. This may increase the affinity of SE-positive *HLA-DRB1* molecules for citrullined peptides.

Several years ago Zanelli et al [25] introduced a new shared epitope located at the same position of the *HLA-DRB1* molecule, as the DERAA positive molecule appeared to be associated with protection against RA. In this hypothesis, replicated in several studies [26, 27], the *HLA-DRB1* DERAA sequence functions not as a part of the p4 pocket of the DRβ1 molecule, but as a peptide that can bind to *HLA-DQ* molecules and then be recognized by regulatory T cells that suppress disease-inducing T cells.

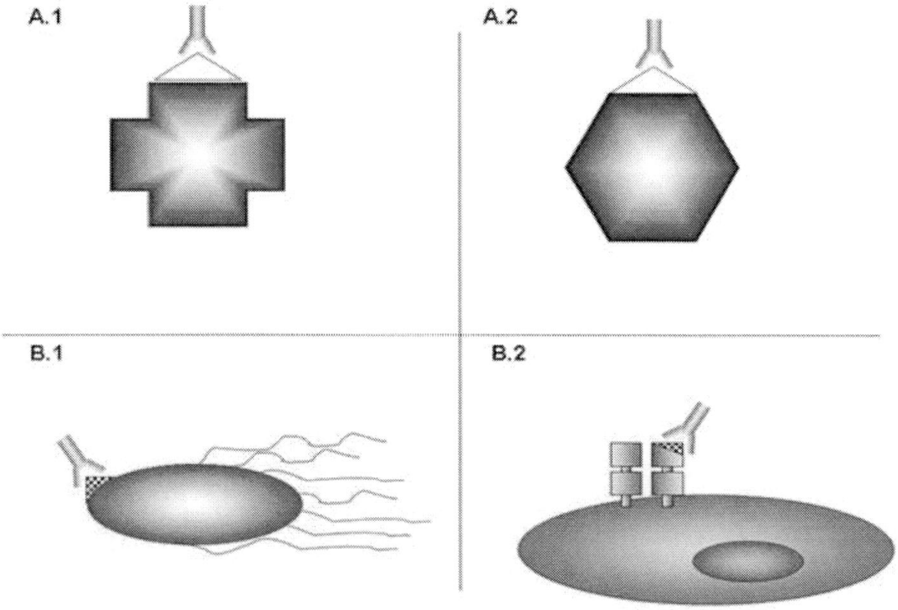

Figure 2. Molecular mimicry:
A) Alpha-Enolase:
A.1.- Antibodies are generated against the microbial alpha-enolase.
A.2.- Antibodies against the microbial alpha-enolases are directed against human alpha-enolase.
B) Proteus:
B.1.-Antibodies are generated against a surface glycoprotein.
B.2.- Antibodies initially directed against the *Proteus sp.* glycoprotein are now directed against the SE peptides from the HLA-DRB1 protein

The contribution of the shared epitope alleles to the total genetic variability of RA ranges from 18 to 37%[20, 28]. However, the SE hypothesis has left questions unanswered [29]. It is unclear whether the MHC *locus* predisposes to RA per se or owing to the development of anti-citrullinated peptide antibodies, which in turn would predispose to RA [3, 30].

The first theories to explain how expression of the shared epitope contributes to RA focus on the concept of "molecular mimicry" or cross-reactivity between bacterial or viral peptides and self antigens. Supposed by, the immune response initially directed at the microbial peptide spreads to tissues presenting the cross-reactive self peptide, in this case specific residues of the HLA molecule itself, resulting in autoimmunity. The sequence identity between the SE and a portion of an Epstein-Barr virus glycoprotein or *Proteus sp.* haemolysin supports this theory [31, 32]. In the same line, the immune response would be initially focused on a microbial enzyme, in this case the cross-reactive self peptide might be the human protein equivalent to the microbial enzyme, and both proteins may share similar residues. An example of this theory is the alpha-enolase; in 2008 a new immunodominant epitope the CEP-1, an epitope from *Porphyromonas gingivalis* alpha-enolase, was described. The generation of antibodies against CEP-1 epitope, results in this case in a cross-reactivity between bacterial and human α-enolase [33].

Current theories focus on the role of the MHC class II molecule in binding specific peptides and presenting them to CD4+ T lymphocytes via recognition by the T cell receptor.

HLA-DRB1 SE alleles could bind citrullinated peptides more strongly. Citrullinated peptides act as self-antigens and are present in the synovial compartment of RA patients. These self-antigens drive B cell maturation and their production of antibodies against citrullinated peptides [34].

Application of Candidate Gene/Region Studies

Different approaches have been used in the past to identify genes associated with RA outside of the MHC. Two decades ago linkage studies led to the identification of chromosomal regions segregating with the disease, but the case-control study is the analysis most used at present.

One effective approach to discovering risk alleles in RA has been the candidate gene approach. At its early stages the selected markers were microsatellites, but soon single nucleotide polymorphisms (SNPs) took their place.

This kind of studies led to the description of the tyrosine-phospatase gene, *PTPN22*, as susceptibility factor for RA [4]. In 2004 Begovich *et al* [4]. performed a case-control association study of 87 putative functional SNPs in RA candidate genes. A missense C to T substitution at nucleotide position 1858 of this gene leads to replacement of triptophan for arginine at residue 620 of the protein product. The resulting gain of function, with enhanced regulation of T-cells to escape clonal deletion, thereby predisposes to autoimmunity. Among individuals of European ancestry, the *PTPN22 locus* continues to be the non MHC region with the strongest effect in RA susceptibility, as estimated by the odds ratio [13].

The discovery of the *STAT4* polymorphism rs7574865 as a susceptibility factor for RA is an example of a combined strategy between linkage and case-control studies. Initially, Remmers *et al* [35]. selected candidate genes from a linkage region of 52 Mb on chromosome 2q, containing the *STAT1* and *STAT4* genes, previously defined by Amos et al [6]. They identified the tag SNPs of this region and performed the corresponding fine mapping. The top associated marker was the one induced by several key cytokines, including interleuking-12 and type 1 interferon, as well as interleukin-23. *STAT4* is a latent cytosolic factor that, after activation by cytokines, is phosporilated and accumulates in the nucleus. STAT4 stimulates transcription of specific genes including interferon-γ, a key indicator of T-cell differentiation into type 1 helper T (Th1) cells. Therefore, STAT4-dependent signalling plays a critical role in the development of a Th1-type T-cell response [5].

The association of a polymorphism located in the cytotoxic T-lymphocyte antigen 4 (*CTLA4*) gene with the development of rheumatoid arthritis had been cause of controversy. After the initial study performed at 1998 that observed a marginal difference between cases and controls [36], several studies had been performed with inconsistent results. After several years a meta-analysis confirmed the association of the SNP rs3087243, which maps to *CTLA4,* with RA development [37].

Expanding List of Known Rheumatoid Arthritis Risk Variants: Genome-Wide Association Studies

Multiple candidate genes were tested for an association with various diseases before the human genome sequence was completed. However, only a limited number of those genes have been replicated.

The genome-wide association studies (GWAS) tried to analyze the whole genome to identify new associated alleles. The first attempt to carry out this kind of analysis was performed in 2005; in this study 27039 microsatellites were used to genotype 375 Japanese RA patients [38].

The analysis of SNPs instead of microsatellites led to an accurate definition of the associated regions. To use this kind of markers in the GWAS the confluence of several factors was necessary. The first of them, of the whole genome was sequenced and the SNP currently present at the human genome where described. To notice, nine out of ten of the described SNPs are highly correlated (r^2>0.80). As a consequence, only a small portion of the SNPs, conformed by tag SNPs, need to be tested directly in a GWAS.

Moreover, the development of new SNP genotyping technologies of high throughput have allowed investigators to screen common variation across the human genome more efficiently [7, 8].

Current GWAS combined this technology with large case-control collections to identify associated alleles. Several associations at *TRAF1-C5*, 6q23, or *REL loci* have been independently described by this kind of analysis [9-12].

The Wellcome Trust Case Control Consortium (WTCCC) performed the first GWAS pointing to an association between the 6q23 region and rheumatoid arthritis [39]. It was replicated at independent studies [10, 11]. In this region, the two independently associated SNPs (rs6920220 and rs10499194) are flanked by two genes, oligodendrocyte lineage transcription factor 3 (*OLIG3*) and TNF-α-induced protein 3 (*TNFAIP3*). *OLIG3* appears to be important in the development and differentiation of neuronal cells, and for the same reason it does not seem to be a good candidate in the development of RA. By contrast, *TNFAIP3* is an attractive candidate gene for RA susceptibility, because it acts as a negative regulator of the transcription factor NF-κB in response to TNF [40].

Several months later *Plenge et al*, [9] analyzed 297,086 SNPs which covered more than 20,000 human genes in a cohort of 1522 anti-CCP positive rheumatoid arthritis patients from the North American Rheumatoid Arthritis Consortium (NARAC) and from the Epidemiological Investigation of Rheumatoid Arthritis (EIRA). They observed a single SNP (rs3764847) within a region on chromosome 9 that maps to the *TRAF1-C5 locus* [9]. *TRAF1* encodes an intracellular protein that acts as a negative regulator of the CD40/NF-κB pathway. The TRAF1 protein binds several intra-cellular proteins including the NF-κB inhibitory protein TNFAIP3 [41, 42].

In 2009 Gregersen *et al.* [12] described the association of the intronic SNP rs13031237G>T in the *REL* gene as a risk factor for rheumatoid arthritis (RA), in an expansion of previous genome-wide association studies. The c-Rel protein is an NF-κB family member that functions to regulate CD40 transcription [43] and recent data indicate that c-Rel promotes the development of Treg progenitors [44].

Moreover, GWAS results can be combined to conduct meta-analysis across multiple studies. Initially, this strategy led to identify five new associations at: *CCL21,* gene encoding for a cytokine that stimulates chemotaxis *in vitro* for thymocytes and activated T cells and inhibits hematopoiesis; *KIF5A,* a member of the kinesin family of proteins, is part of a multisubunit complex that has been implicated in intracellular organelle transport; *CD40* is a receptor of the TNF family involved on a broad variety of immune responses, including mebmory B cell development; *PRKCQ* , codes for a member of the protein kinase C family, is a calcium independent protein involved in T cell activation through the activation of the transcriptor factors NF-κB and AP-1; *TNFRSF14,* which encodes for a member of the TNF-receptor superfamily, at the beginning it was identified as mediator of herpes simplex virus entry and this protein also binds several *TRAF* family members [40, 45].

The last attempt to identify new rheumatoid arthritis risk markers was a GWAS meta-analysis of 5539 cases and 20169 controls, with a replication in 6768 RA patients and 8806 healthy controls. At this study, the authors support the RA risk *loci* previously identified among individuals of European ancestry and identify 7 new risk *loci*, summarized in table 1 [46].

Table 1. Known Snps Associated With Rheumatoid Arthritis Risk In Caucasian Individuals

Gene(s)	Associated Id	*Locus*	Gene(s)	Associated Id	*Locus*
TNFRSF14	rs3890745	1p36	*HLA-DRB1*	rs6910071	6p21
PTPN22	rs2476601	1p13	*PRDM1*	rs548234	6q21
CD2/CD58	rs11586238	1p13	*TNFAIP3*	rs10499194	6q23
FCGR2A	rs12746613	1q23		rs6920220	
PTPRC	rs10919563	1q31		rs5029937	
SPRED2	rs937434	2p14	*TAGAP*	rs394581	6q25
REL	rs13031237	2p16	*IRF5*	rs10488631	7q32
AFF3	rs11676922	2q11	*BLK*	rs2736340	8p23
	rs10865035		*CCL21*	rs951005	9p13
STAT4	rs7574865	2q32		rs2812378	
CD28	rs1980422	2q33	*TRAF1/C5*	rs3761847	9q33
CTLA4	rs3087243	2q33	*IL2RA*	rs706778	10p15
PXK	rs13315591	3p14		rs2104286	
RBPJ	rs8740400	4p15	*PRKCQ*	rs4750316	10p15
IL2/IL21	rs6822844	4q27	*TRAF6*	rs540386	11p12
ANKRD55/IL6ST	rs6859219	5q11	*KIF5A/PIP4K2C*	rs1678542	12q13
C5orf30	rs26232	5q21	*CD40*	rs4810485	20q13
CCR6	rs3093023	6q27	*IL2RB*	rs3218253	22q12

At present, approximately half of the genetic susceptibility to RA remains to be explained. Additional susceptibility *loci* may exist in regions of the genome that are not well covered by the whole-genome chip arrays. Alternatively, rare variants or genomic rearrangements may contribute to susceptibility, but to date, these have not been extensively examined in complex diseases such as RA [3, 13].

Subsets of Disease

The phenotype for multifactorial diseases such as RA is often defined through consensus procedures. As it is the case with most complex disorders large variation in the phenotype of the pathology is observed. Traditionally, RA patients have been classified by the presence or absence of autoantibody response. First they were separated by rheumatoid factor status, but more recently, investigators have focused on the presence of antibodies directed against cyclic citrullinated peptides (anti-CCPs). Since the identification of anti-CCPs antibodies, several studies have confirmed a significant association between the *HLA-DRB1* SE alleles and the presence of anti-CCP antibodies [34, 47, 48].

Other studies correlate genetic polymorphisms with the presence of anti-CCP antibodies. In 2007 Cha *et al.* [49] observed that a *PADI4* haplotype was associated with increased anti-CCP antibodies levels in early RA patients[50]. There is a significant association between the *PTPN22* and the presence of anti-CCP antibodies, too [51].

All the GWAS to date have been biased towards anti-CCP antibodies positive RA patients[9, 10, 40, 52]. For this reason, it is clear that many validated RA risk alleles are more strongly associated with this subgroup. It will be of particular interest to perform these GWAS in collections of anti-CCP antibodies negative RA patients.

Ethnic Differences

Most genetic studies in RA have been carried out in populations of European ancestry and show remarkable consistency in findings across those populations. Nonetheless, substantial differences in genetic RA susceptibility factors have been found between European and Asian populations [53, 54].

The MHC region is the most heterogeneous region in the human genome. Various studies have studied the associations with the *HLA-DRB1* genes, and multiple ethnic groups have found alleles of the *HLA-DRB1* gene associated with susceptibility to RA [55]. The prevalence of shared epitope alleles is likely to present important variations in different ethnic groups. For example in Native Americans the most prevalent *HLA-DRB1* allele is the *HLA-DRB1*1402* [14], *the HLA-DRB1*0102* is the most prevalent allele in African populations [16]. Nevertheless, the vast majority of the studies confirm a significant increase in the frequency of alleles containing the shared epitope in RA patients compared to healthy controls [18].

PTPN22 polymorphisms have been identified in European populations, but are rarely found in Asian populations [53, 54]. Another example of heterogeneity is that polymorphisms at 6q23 are non-polymorphic at Asian populations [54]. By contrast, the *PADI4* gene is associated in multiple Asian populations, but it does not appear to be associated with RA in Caucasians [53]. The same situation is found with *FCLR3* and *SLC22A4* genes, which have been shown to be associated with RA in Asian but not Caucasian populations [54].

Other susceptibility *loci,* such as *STAT4,* are replicated in Asian an European descendent, but not in African Americans [56].

These data indicate that most of the disease-associated variants have arisen independently in different continental populations and that different points in disease-associated pathways are influenced by genetic risk factors in the different populations [54].

One would expect that GWAS in non-European descent populations would reveal different susceptibility *loci* than those described in Caucasian GWAS.

Implicated Pathways in Rheumatoid Arthritis Risk?

Several of the genes described above are implicated in the CD40/NF-κB pathway. So it seems that this pathway has to be involved in the development of RA. Before the role of each gene/protein could be ascribed, two ideas must be considered. First, when a risk polymorphism is identified, it is often assigned to a gene which maps next to it, but it does not mean that the genetic marker influences the gene expression by itself. Usually the gene with a putative biological role is chosen, but it might be implicated at the disease or not [13]. Second, the reported allele is not necessarily the causal one, it may represent a highly correlated proxy for an unidentified causal allele [13].

Several genes at the CD40/NF-κB pathway, described not only through genetic studies but also by functional ones, are related with the development of RA [43]. The *CD40* gene was identified in a meta-analysis of GWAS [57], CD40 is a TNF receptor family member that acts as costimulator in T-cells. Functional studies showed that CD40 signalling is necessary for the activation of B cells and the production of antibodies, since $CD40^-$ deficient mice do not develop arthritis [58]. Other gene related with this pathway is *TNFRSF14*, a member of the TNF receptor superfamily, which encodes a protein that has been shown to bind TRAF family members including TRAF1. The *TNFAIP3* gene encodes a cytoplasmic zinc finger protein, A20, an inhibitor of NF-kB activation. A20-deficent mices show a sustained NF-kB response and severe inflammation [59]. Both *TNFAIP3* and *TRAF1* act as negative regulators of the CD40/NF-kB pathway [60]. The last *locus* found associated with this pathway was *REL*, an NF-kB family member that functions to regulate transcription of CD40. Recent data suggest that CD40 and c-Rel proteins physically interact, forming a heterodimer that translocates to the nucleus and regulates the transcriptional activity of c-Rel target genes, such as *CD154*, *BLyS/BAFF* and *Bfl-1A1* [43].

NF-kB, a protein complex that acts as a transcription factor, is found in almost all cell types and it is involved in a variety of cellular responses to stimuli. Both TNF and CD40 signal through NF-kB to exert their effects on the immune system. As shown in Figure 3, several of the RA risk *loci* contain genes that are involved in NF-kB signalling, including the above mentioned *CD40, TRAF1, TNFAIP3, TNFRSF14* and *REL* [13].

Common Variants/Multiple Diseases

Nowadays some authors believe that in autoimmune diseases like RA, disease genes may not be disease specific. This theory called "*common variants/Multiple diseases*" is based on the familiar aggregation effect observed and the existence of common genetic markers associated with the development of several autoimmune diseases[61-63].

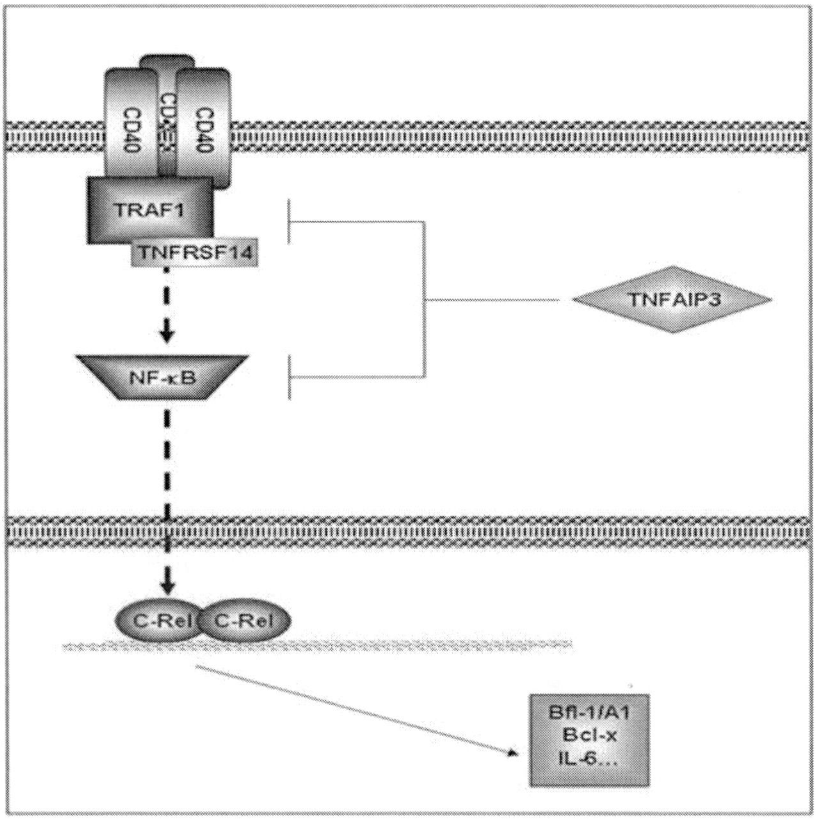

Figure 3. CD40/NF-κB signal pathway. The scheme shows the proteins from RA risk *loci* genes

Structural Variants

GWAS have been extremely successful in associating SNPs with susceptibility to common diseases, but published SNPs associations account for only a fraction of the genetic component of RA. A recent study performed to detect the "missing heritability" of rheumatoid arthritis used an array of copy number variations (CNV) to type 2000 RA and 3000 controls. They concluded that common CNVs typable on current platforms are unlikely to have a major role in the genetic basis of RA [64].

The next step to detect the "missing heritability" for RA could be to analyze genomic rearrangements such as inversions and translocations.

Take-Home Messages

Although much of the recent excitement in the field has resulted from the utilization of GWAS to search for genes outside the MHC, the single most important contribution to genetic risk for RA clearly resides within the MHC.

Validated non-MHC RA risk alleles explain about 23% of the genetic weight of disease, indicating that additional alleles remains to be discovered [46].

GWAS have been performed with European ancestry cohorts, so it will be of particular interest to perform these GWAS in collections of non-European ancestry.

References

[1] MacGregor, AJ; Snieder, H; Rigby, AS; Koskenvuo, M; Kaprio, J; Aho, K; *et al.* Characterizing the quantitative genetic contribution to rheumatoid arthritis using data from twins. *Arthritis Rheum*, 2000, 43, 30-7.

[2] Gregersen, PK; Silver, J; Winchester, RJ. The shared epitope hypothesis. An approach to understanding the molecular genetics of susceptibility to rheumatoid arthritis. *Arthritis Rheum.,* 1987, 30, 1205-13.

[3] Barton, A; Worthington, J. Genetic susceptibility to rheumatoid arthritis: an emerging picture. *Arthritis Rheum.,* 2009, 61, 1441-6.

[4] Begovich, AB; Carlton, VE; Honigberg, LA; Schrodi, SJ; Chokkalingam, AP; Alexander, HC; *et al.* A missense single-nucleotide polymorphism in a gene encoding a protein tyrosine phosphatase (PTPN22) is associated with rheumatoid arthritis. *Am J Hum Genet*, 2004, 75, 330-7.

[5] Remmers, EF; Plenge, RM; Lee, AT; Graham, RR; Hom, G; Behrens, TW; *et al.* STAT4 and the risk of rheumatoid arthritis and systemic lupus erythematosus. *N Engl J Med.,* 2007, 357, 977-86.

[6] Amos, CI; Chen, WV; Lee, A; Li, W; Kern, M; Lundsten, R; *et al.* High-density SNP analysis of 642 Caucasian families with rheumatoid arthritis identifies two new linkage regions on 11p12 and 2q33. *Genes Immun*, 2006, 7, 277-86.

[7] Shen, F; Huang, J; Fitch, KR; Truong, VB; Kirby, A; Chen, W; *et al.* Improved detection of global copy number variation using high density; non-polymorphic oligonucleotide probes. *BMC Genet*, 2008, 9, 27.

[8] Bhangale, TR; Rieder, MJ; Nickerson, DA. Estimating coverage and power for genetic association studies using near-complete variation data. *Nat Genet*, 2008, 40, 841-3.

[9] Plenge, RM; Seielstad, M; Padyukov, L; Lee, AT; Remmers, EF; Ding, B; *et al.* TRAF1-C5 as a risk locus for rheumatoid arthritis--a genomewide study. *N Engl J Med.,* 2007, 357, 1199-209.

[10] Thomson, W; Barton, A; Ke, X; Eyre, S; Hinks, A; Bowes, J; *et al.* Rheumatoid arthritis association at 6q23. *Nat Genet*, 2007, 39, 1431-3.

[11] Plenge, RM; Cotsapas, C; Davies, L; Price, AL; de Bakker, PI; Maller, J; *et al.* Two independent alleles at 6q23 associated with risk of rheumatoid arthritis. *Nat Genet*, 2007, 39, 1477-82.

[12] Gregersen, PK; Amos, CI; Lee, AT; Lu, Y; Remmers, EF; Kastner, DL; *et al.* REL; encoding a member of the NF-kappaB family of transcription factors; is a newly defined risk locus for rheumatoid arthritis. *Nat Genet*, 2009, 41, 820-3.

[13] Plenge, RM. Recent progress in rheumatoid arthritis genetics: one step towards improved patient care. *Curr Opin Rheumatol,* 2009, 21, 262-71.

[14] Del Puente, A; Knowler, WC; Pettitt, DJ; Bennett, PH. High incidence and prevalence of rheumatoid arthritis in Pima Indians. *Am J Epidemiol*, 1989, 129, 1170-8.

[15] Alamanos, Y; Drosos, AA. Epidemiology of adult rheumatoid arthritis. *Autoimmun Rev*, 2005, 4, 130-6.

[16] Silman, AJ; Ollier, W; Holligan, S; Birrell, F; Adebajo, A; Asuzu, MC; *et al.* Absence of rheumatoid arthritis in a rural Nigerian population. J Rheumatol 1993, 20, 618-22.

[17] Alamanos, Y; Voulgari, PV; Drosos, AA. Incidence and prevalence of rheumatoid arthritis; based on the 1987 American College of Rheumatology criteria: a systematic review. *Semin Arthritis Rheum.,* 2006, 36, 182-8.

[18] Tobon, GJ; Youinou, P; Saraux, A. The environment; geo-epidemiology; and autoimmune disease: Rheumatoid arthritis. *Autoimmun Rev*; 9, A288-92.

[19] Dieude, P. Rheumatic diseases: environment and genetics. *Joint Bone Spine*, 2009, 76, 602-7.

[20] Deighton, CM; Walker, DJ; Griffiths, ID; Roberts DF. The contribution of HLA to rheumatoid arthritis. *Clin Genet*, 1989, 36, 178-82.

[21] Risch, N. Linkage strategies for genetically complex traits. I. Multilocus models. *Am J Hum Genet,* 1990, 46, 222-8.

[22] del Junco, D; Luthra, HS; Annegers, JF; Worthington, JW; Kurland, LT. The familial aggregation of rheumatoid arthritis and its relationship to the HLA-DR4 association. *Am J Epidemiol,* 1984, 119, 813-29.

[23] Stastny, P; Fink, CW. HLA-Dw4 in adult and juvenile rheumatoid arthritis. *Transplant Proc*, 1977, 9, 1863-6.

[24] Dessen, A; Lawrence, CM; Cupo, S; Zaller, DM; Wiley, DC. X-ray crystal structure of HLA-DR4 (DRA*0101, DRB1*0401) complexed with a peptide from human collagen II. *Immunity*, 1997, 7, 473-81.

[25] Zanelli, E; Vos, K; Breedveld, F; de Vries, R; David, C. Role of HLA-DQ in rheumatoid arthritis susceptibility: comment on the article by de Vries et al. *Arthritis Rheum.,* 2000, 43, 946-8.

[26] van der Horst-Bruinsma, IE; Visser, H; Hazes, JM; Breedveld, FC; Verduyn, W; Schreuder, GM; et al. HLA-DQ-associated predisposition to and dominant HLA-DR-associated protection against rheumatoid arthritis. *Hum Immunol*, 1999, 60, 152-8.

[27] van der Helm-van Mil, AH; Huizinga, TW; Schreuder, GM; Breedveld, FC; de Vries, RR; Toes, RE. An independent role of protective HLA class II alleles in rheumatoid arthritis severity and susceptibility. *Arthritis Rheum.,* 2005, 52, 2637-44.

[28] van der Woude, D; Huizinga, TW. Every shared epitope allele for itself? *Nat Rev Rheumatol*, 2009, 5, 477-8.

[29] Suzuki, A; Yamada, R; Chang, X; Tokuhiro, S; Sawada, T; Suzuki, M; et al. Functional haplotypes of PADI4, encoding citrullinating enzyme peptidylarginine deiminase 4, are associated with rheumatoid arthritis. *Nat Genet*, 2003, 34, 395-402.

[30] Varade, J; Loza-Santamaria, E; Fernandez-Arquero, M; Lamas, JR; de Los Angeles Figueredo, M; Jover, JA; et al. Shared epitope and anti-cyclic citrullinated peptide antibodies: relationship with age at onset and duration of disease in rheumatoid arthritis. *J Rheumatol*, 2009, 36, 1085-6.

[31] Munz, C; Lunemann, JD; Getts, MT; Miller, SD. Antiviral immune responses: triggers of or triggered by autoimmunity? *Nat Rev Immunol*, 2009, 9, 246-58.

[32] Ebringer, A; Rashid, T; Wilson, C. Rheumatoid arthritis; Proteus; anti-CCP antibodies and Karl Popper. *Autoimmun Rev*, 2010, 9, 216-23.

[33] Mahdi, H; Fisher, BA; Kallberg, H; Plant, D; Malmstrom, V; Ronnelid, J; et al. Specific interaction between genotype; smoking and autoimmunity to citrullinated alpha-enolase in the etiology of rheumatoid arthritis. *Nat Genet*, 2009, 41, 1319-24.

[34] Van Gaalen, FA; van Aken, J; Huizinga, TW; Schreuder, GM; Breedveld, FC; Zanelli, E*; et al.* Association between HLA class II genes and autoantibodies to cyclic citrullinated peptides (CCPs) influences the severity of rheumatoid arthritis. *Arthritis Rheum.,* 2004, 50, 2113-21.

[35] Korman, BD; Kastner, DL; Gregersen, PK; Remmers, EF; Taylor, KE; Remmers, EF; et al. STAT4, genetics; mechanisms; and implications for autoimmunity. *Curr Allergy Asthma Rep*, 2008, 8, 398-403.

[36] Seidl, C; Donner, H; Fischer, B; Usadel, KH; Seifried, E; Kaltwasser, JP; et al. CTLA4 codon 17 dimorphism in patients with rheumatoid arthritis. *Tissue Antigens*, 1998, 51, 62-6.

[37] Daha, NA; Kurreeman, FA; Marques, RB; Stoeken-Rijsbergen, G; Verduijn, W; Huizinga, TW; et al. Confirmation of STAT4, IL2/IL21, and CTLA4 polymorphisms in rheumatoid arthritis. *Arthritis Rheum.,* 2009, 60, 1255-60.

[38] Tamiya, G; Shinya, M; Imanishi, T; Ikuta, T; Makino, S; Okamoto, K; et al. Whole genome association study of rheumatoid arthritis using 27 039 microsatellites. *Hum Mol Genet*, 2005, 14, 2305-21.

[39] Genome-wide association study of 14, 000 cases of seven common diseases and 3, 000 shared controls. *Nature*, 2007, 447, 661-78.

[40] Barton, A; Thomson, W; Ke, X; Eyre, S; Hinks, A; Bowes, J*; et al.* Rheumatoid arthritis susceptibility *loci at chromosomes*, 10p15, 12q13 and 22q13. *Nat Genet*, 2008, 40, 1156-9.

[41] Firestein, GS. Evolving concepts of rheumatoid arthritis. *Nature*, 2003, 423, 356-61.

[42] Bradley, JR; Pober, JS. Tumor necrosis factor receptor-associated factors (TRAFs). *Oncogene*, 2001, 20, 6482-91.

[43] Criswell, LA. Gene discovery in rheumatoid arthritis highlights the CD40/NF-kappaB signaling pathway in disease pathogenesis. *Immunol Rev*, 233, 55-61.

[44] Vang, KB; Yang, J; Pagan, AJ; Li, LX; Wang, J; Green, JM; et al. Cutting edge: CD28 and c-Rel-dependent pathways initiate regulatory T cell development. *J Immunol*, 184, 4074-7.

[45] Raychaudhuri, S. Recent advances in the genetics of rheumatoid arthritis. *Curr Opin Rheumatol*, 22, 109-18.

[46] Stahl, EA; Raychaudhuri, S; Remmers, EF; Xie, G; Eyre, S; Thomson, BP; et al. Genome-wide association study meta-analysis identifies seven new rheumatoid arthritis risk loci. Nat Genet.

[47] Huizinga, TW; Amos, CI; van der Helm-van Mil, AH; Chen, W; van Gaalen, FA; Jawaheer, D; et al. Refining the complex rheumatoid arthritis phenotype based on specificity of the HLA-DRB1 shared epitope for antibodies to citrullinated proteins. *Arthritis Rheum.,* 2005, 52, 3433-8.

[48] Berglin, E; Padyukov, L; Sundin, U; Hallmans, G; Stenlund, H; Van Venrooij, WJ; et al. A combination of autoantibodies to cyclic citrullinated peptide (CCP) and HLA-

DRB1 locus antigens is strongly associated with future onset of rheumatoid arthritis. *Arthritis Res Ther*, 2004, 6, R303-8.

[49] Cha, S; Choi, CB; Han, TU; Kang, CP; Kang, C; Bae, SC. Association of anti-cyclic citrullinated peptide antibody levels with PADI4 haplotypes in early rheumatoid arthritis and with shared epitope alleles in very late rheumatoid arthritis. *Arthritis Rheum.,* 2007, 56, 1454-63.

[50] Barton, A; Bowes, J; Eyre, S; Symmons, D; Worthington, J; Silman, A. Investigation of polymorphisms in the PADI4 gene in determining severity of inflammatory polyarthritis. *Ann Rheum Dis*, 2005, 64, 1311-5.

[51] Johansson, M; Arlestig, L; Hallmans, G; Rantapaa-Dahlqvist, S. PTPN22 polymorphism and anti-cyclic citrullinated peptide antibodies in combination strongly predicts future onset of rheumatoid arthritis and has a specificity of 100% for the disease. *Arthritis Res Ther*, 2006, 8, R19.

[52] Raychaudhuri, S; Thomson, BP; Remmers, EF; Eyre, S; Hinks, A; Guiducci, C; et al. Genetic variants at CD28, PRDM1 and CD2/CD58 are associated with rheumatoid arthritis risk. *Nat Genet*, 2009, 41, 1313-8.

[53] Kochi, Y; Suzuki, A; Yamada, R; Yamamoto, K. Genetics of rheumatoid arthritis: underlying evidence of ethnic differences. *J Autoimmun*, 2009, 32, 158-62.

[54] Lee, HS; Korman, BD; Le, JM; Kastner, DL; Remmers, EF; Gregersen, PK; et al. Genetic risk factors for rheumatoid arthritis differ in Caucasian and Korean populations. *Arthritis Rheum.,* 2009, 60, 364-71.

[55] Gonzalez-Gay, MA; Garcia-Porrua, C; Hajeer, AH. Influence of human leukocyte antigen-DRB1 on the susceptibility and severity of rheumatoid arthritis. *Semin Arthritis Rheum.,* 2002, 31, 355-60.

[56] Kelley, JM; Hughes, LB; Malik, A; Danila, MI; Edberg, Y; Alarcon, GS; et al. Genetic variants of STAT4 associated with rheumatoid arthritis in persons of Asian and European ancestry do not replicate in African Americans. *Ann Rheum Dis*, 69, 625-6.

[57] Raychaudhuri, S; Remmers, EF; Lee, AT; Hackett, R; Guiducci, C; Burtt, NP; et al. Common variants at CD40 and other loci confer risk of rheumatoid arthritis. *Nat Genet*, 2008, 40, 1216-23.

[58] Kyburz, D; Carson, DA; Corr, M. The role of CD40 ligand and tumor necrosis factor alpha signaling in the transgenic K/BxN mouse model of rheumatoid arthritis. *Arthritis Rheum.,* 2000, 43, 2571-7.

[59] Lee, EG; Boone, DL; Chai, S; Libby, SL; Chien, M; Lodolce, JP; et al. Failure to regulate TNF-induced NF-kappaB and cell death responses in A20-deficient mice. *Science*, 2000, 289, 2350-4.

[60] Bishop, GA. The multifaceted roles of TRAFs in the regulation of B-cell function. *Nat Rev Immunol*, 2004, 4, 775-86.

[61] Becker, KG. The common variants/multiple disease hypothesis of common complex genetic disorders. *Med Hypotheses*, 2004, 62, 309-17.

[62] Martinez, A; Varade, J; Marquez, A; Cenit, MC; Espino, L; Perdigones, N; et al., Association of the STAT4 gene with increased susceptibility for some immune-mediated diseases. *Arthritis Rheum.,* 2008, 58, 2598-602.

[63] Kurreeman, FA; Goulielmos, GN; Alizadeh, BZ; Rueda, B; Houwing-Duistermaat, J; Sanchez, E*; et al.* The TRAF1-C5 region on chromosome 9q33 is associated with multiple autoimmune diseases. *Ann Rheum Dis*, 69, 696-9.

[64] Wellcome_Trust_Case_Control_Consortium. Genome-wide association study of CNVs in 16, 000 cases of eight common diseases and 3, 000 shared controls. *Nature*, 2010, 464, 713-20.

In: Rheumatoid Arthritis: Prevalence, Risk... ISBN: 978-1-61761-931-1
Editor: Michael H. Madsen

Chapter 5

Long-Term Results of Computer-Assisted Cervical Reconstruction for Cervical Disorders in Rheumatoid Arthritis

Jun Takahashi* and Hiroyuki Kato
Department of Orthopaedic Surgery, Shinshu University,
School of Medicine, Nagano, Japan

Abstract

To reconstruct highly destructed unstable rheumatoid arthritis (RA) cervical lesions, the authors have been using C1/2 transarticular and cervical pedicle screw fixations. Pedicle screw fixation and C1/2 transarticular screw fixation are biomechanically superior to other fixation techniques for RA patients. However, due to severe spinal deformity and small anatomical size of the vertebra, including the lateral mass and pedicle, in the most RA cervical lesions, these screw fixation procedures are technically demanding and pose the potential risk of neurovascular injuries. The purpose of this study was to evaluate the long-term results of cervical reconstruction for the deformed, fragile, and small RA spine lesions using computer-assisted image-guidance systems. A frameless, stereotactic image-guidance system that is CT-based, and optoelectronic was used for correct screw placement. A total of 20 patients (14 females, 6 males) with cervical disorders due to RA were surgically treated using the image-guidance system.

Postoperative computerized tomography was used to determine the accuracy of the screw placement. Neural and vascular complications associated with screw insertion and postoperative neural recovery were evaluated. Postoperative radiological evaluations

* Corresponding author: E-mail: jtaka@shinshu-u.ac.jp, Department of Orthopaedic Surgery, Shinshu University, School of Medicine 3-1-1 Asahi, Matsumoto-City, Nagano 390-8621, Japan FAX: 81-263-35-8844 Phone: 81-263-37-2659

revealed that only 1 (2.5%; C4) of 40 screws inserted into the cervical pedicle had perforated more than 50% of the screw diameter (critical breach). However, no neurovascular complications were observed. According to Ranawat's classification, 8 patients remained the same, 11 patients showed improvement, and 1 patient showed deterioration. Instrumentation failure, loss of reduction, or nonunion was not observed at the final follow-up (average 49 months; range 24–108 months). In this study, the authors demonstrated that image-guidance systems could be applied safely to the cervical lesions caused by RA. Image-guidance systems are useful tools in preoperative planning and in transarticular or transpedicular screw placement in the cervical spine of RA patients.

Keywords: Cervical spine, Image guidance, Rheumatoid arthritis, Cervical pedicle screw, Transarticular screw

Introduction

There are various cervical disorders caused by rheumatoid arthritis (RA). The most common disorders include atrantoaxial (C1/2) instability and subluxation in the mid- and lower-cervical spine [1,2]. These conditions sometimes cause myelopathy, severe pain, or both, either of which impairs the quality of life of RA patients [3]. In such cases, reconstruction surgery may be indicated. Posterior procedures using sublaminar wiring or hook systems have been employed; however, these sometimes result in loss of reduction and/or nonunion [4, 5]. Innovative methods such as C1/2 transarticular and cervical pedicle screw techniques provide greater biomechanical stability compared to conventional posterior fusion techniques [6, 7]. Jones et al. [8] reported that cervical pedicle screws have a significantly higher resistance to pull-out forces than lateral mass screws. However, due to severe spinal deformity and small anatomical size of the vertebra including the lateral mass and pedicle in most of the RA cervical lesions, these screw fixation procedures are technically demanding and pose the potential risk of neurovascular injuries [9-11].

Frameless stereotactic technology was first designed for intra-cranial surgery for guidance of unseen lesions [12]. Computer-assisted techniques were introduced in spine surgery in the 1990s to improve accuracy and safety of operative procedures [13,14]. CT-based optoelectronic navigation was originally introduced by Nolte et al. [14]. Amiot et al. [13] later performed this technique in vitro with a magnetic-field based navigator, however this never really gained clinical acceptance. Laine et al. [15] presented evidence for improvement of accuracy under clinical conditions using this technique. In 1996, we started the laboratory testing and the clinical application of computer-assisted spine surgery [16-21]. The purpose of this study was to evaluate the long-term results of cervical reconstruction for the deformed, fragile, and small RA spine lesions using computer-assisted image-guidance systems.

Materials and Methods

Between January 2000 and January 2007, a total of 20 patients (14 females, 6 males) with cervical disorders due to RA were surgically treated using the image-guidance system. The mean age at the time of surgery was 62 years (range 51–80 years). The cervical disorders were atlanto-axial subluxation (AAS) in six cases, AAS and vertical subluxation of the atlas (VS) in six, subaxial subluxation (SAS) in two and AAS + VS + SAS in six. According to Ranawat's classification [19], the neurological deficits were class 2 in seven cases, class 3A in six, and class 3B in seven. The Ranawat's classification is defined as follows; class 1, no neural deficit; class 2, subjective weakness with hyper-reflexia and dysesthesia; class 3A, objective findings of paresis and long-tract signs, but ambulation possible; class 3B, quadriparesis with resultant inability to walk or to feed oneself.

Navigation and Surgical Procedures

A frameless stereotactic image-guidance system (Stealth Station and Stealth Station TREONTM; Medtronic, Sofamor Danek, Memphis, TN, USA) was used for correct screw placement and fixation of the cervical spine. The basic data used for navigation were preoperative CT scan imaging data, consisting of consecutive axial slices, 1 mm in thickness of the cervical spine of the RA patients. The data were transferred to the system computer and were reconstructed into two-dimensional (2-D) and three-dimensional (3-D) images on a video monitor. Other mechanical components consisted of a computer workstation, a surgical reference frame, a probe rod to indicate the position in the surgical field, infrared light-emitting diodes (LEDs) that were attached to the probe rod, an electro-optical camera as a position sensor connected to the computer, and a drill guide. Infrared beams were tracked by the electro-optical camera system and the position of the respective LEDs was identified in real time in the surgical field.

Registration was performed in order to accurately match the computer-reconstructed 3-D surgical space with the real surgical space, by identifying four or more points on the vertebrae and the corresponding points of the vertebrae on the 3-D CT image on the monitor (matched-pair point registration). Though more precise matching of the two spaces is usually obtained by repeated registration procedures with 30 or more randomized points indicated by the probe on the surface of the vertebral body (surface registration), this group's procedure employs only five to six registration points for two consecutive lamina, to shorten the surgical time. More accurate positioning is possible by using the top of the spinous process and bilateral inferior facet caudal tip as points.

We established a surgical plan a day before surgery and confirmed insertion point of screws, applicability of 3.5 mm screws, point-for-point registration, plus in Magerl's screw procedure, screw position in relation to vertebral artery. This planning procedure took 20– 40 min. Evaluation during the surgical plan for navigation provides further benefit by identifying pedicles with insertion risks and excluding such pedicles from operation (about 10% of all pedicles were excluded). Then, the entrance holes, direction, diameter, and depth of the screws were depicted with a cursor on the monitor, and the surgery was initiated. After exposure of the posterior bony elements of the spine, the reference frame was fixed to the spinous processes and the registration procedures described above were performed. After completion of the registration by matched-pair point and surface registration, the screws were inserted under the guidance of the navigation system. The position of the probe or drill guide was superimposed in real-time on CT images on the monitor, and the screws were introduced into the pedicles at the planned position indicated on the monitor (Figure 1). The required time between fixation of reference frame to spinous process and insertion of pedicle screw to each segment (1 or 2 vertebrae) was 10–15 min. After all screws were set, the reference frame for registration was removed and additional surgical procedures including decompression or bone graft were followed. If pedicle screw insertion was ineligible, sublaminar cable fixation by a high-molecular weight polyethylene cable was performed.

The following surgical procedures were performed with the aid of image-guidance systems: C1/2 transarticular screw (Trans Bone Screw; KiscoMedica, St Priest, France in two patients, and UCSS; Medtronic, Sofamor Danek, Memphis, TN, USA in four patients) fixation (Magerl's procedure [22]) in six patients, cervicothoracic fusion using transpedicular screws (Cervical Pedicle Screw System; Depuy Spine, Inc., Raynham, MA, USA) in two patients, occipitocervical or occipitothoracic fusion using the Olerud cervical system (Nord Opedic, Askim, Sweden) in four patients, and RRS Loop Spinal System (Robert Leid, Tokyo, Japan) in eight patients. All patients had autogenous iliac bone grafts. Patients were permitted to stand and walk from the day after the operation without a collar, since pedicle screw fixation provided enough stability to ambulate without it.

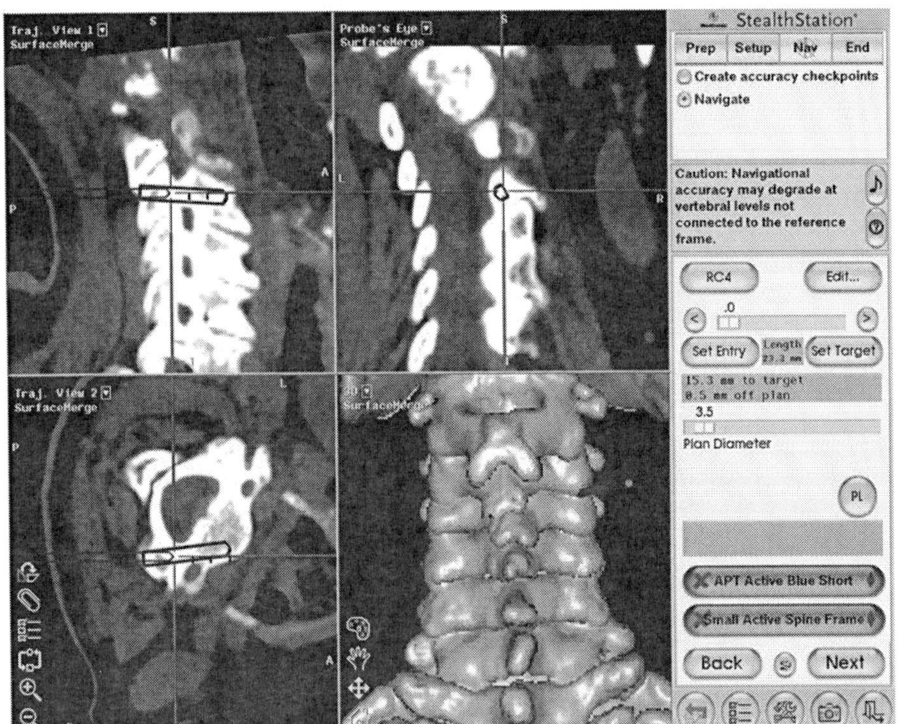

Figure 1. Computer display shown at surgery. The position of the device and surgical plan are shown in four views. The narrow gray arrow indicates the position and direction of the device, and the wide black arrow indicates the planned screw trajectory

X-Ray Assessment

All patients underwent plain a.p. and lateral X-ray films and reconstruction computed tomography (CT) scans of instrumented levels before and after surgery.

Roentgenological measurement of atlantodental interval (ADI) was performed in 18 cases that were accompanied with AAS. Ranawat value was measured using the lateral X-ray image in 18 cases that were not SAS cases [23]. Pedicle screw positions evaluated by CT after surgery were classified as follows; Grade 1: correctly inserted in the pedicle, Grade 2: perforation within 50% of the screw diameter, or Grade 3: perforation more than 50% of the screw diameter. Bony union was evaluated using dynamic X-ray and reconstruction CT sans.

Student's *t*-test using Statcel 2nd edition (OMS publishing Inc., Saitama, Japan) was used for statistical analysis, with $p<0.05$ defined as significant.

Results

A total of 65 screws, including twelve C1/2 transarticular screws and 53 transpedicular screws (C2; 9 screws, C3; 9, C4; 4, C5; 2, C6; 6, C7; 10, T1; 9, T2; 4), were inserted using image-guidance system and resulted in 59, 5, and 1 cases of Grade 1, 2, and 3, respectively. Grade 3 was seen in C4 pedicle and Grade 2 was seen in C3 (2 cases), C4 (1 case) and C6 pedicle (2 case), respectively (Figure 2). The perforation rate of cervical pedicle screws was 2.5% (1/40) when Grade 3 was defined as major perforation. The perforation rate of all screws was 1.5% (1/65).

Eighteen of 20 cases were accompanied with AAS, for which mean ADI values were as follows: before surgery, 6.7±3.5 mm; immediately after surgery, 3.8±1.4 mm; at the final follow-up, 4.6±2.2 mm. Mean ADI value immediately after surgery was significantly small ($p = 0.004$) and was maintained to the final follow-up ($p= 0.04$). VS was shown in 12 of 20 cases, for which mean Ranawat values were as follows: before surgery, 10.1±4.7 mm; immediately after surgery, 11.1±3.4 mm; at the final follow-up, 10.9±3.7 mm. Mean Ranawat value did not show significant change.

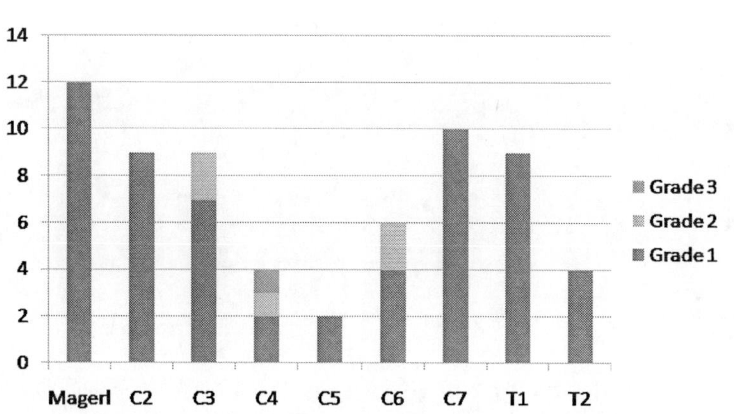

Figure 2. Grade 3 was seen in C4 pedicle and Grade 2 was seen in C3 (2 cases), C4 (1 case), and C6 pedicle (2 cases)

Average operative time was 255 min (range 126–505 min) and the average intraoperative blood loss was 351 ml (range 180–600 ml). According to Ranawat's classification, 8 patients remained the same (2→2; 5 patients, 3A→3A; 1, 3B→3B; 2) and 11 patients showed improvement (2→1; 2 patients, 3A→2; 4, 3B→3A; 5). One patient remained the same (3A→3A) one year after surgery; however, this patient showed deterioration (3A→3B) at final follow-up. Five of the seven patients who could not walk (3B) before surgery could walk (3A) post surgery. Nineteen of the twenty patients maintained the improved ADL level throughout the postoperative course. No instrumentation failure, loss of reduction, or nonunion had occurred at the final follow-up (average 49 months; range 24–108 months). Bony fusion was defined as an absence of segmental motion in functional lateral X-rays with presence of solid bony union observed in reconstruction CT. Solid union was achieved in all 20 patients.

Case Presentations

This patient was a 68-year-old man with non-reducible AAS and VS (Figure 3). In preoperative planning, the authors judged that it was not possible to insert the pedicle screw into the C2pedicles. The following procedures were performed using the navigation system: C1 laminectomy, insertion of bilateral C3 pedicle screw (RRS Loop Spinal System; Robert Leid, Tokyo, Japan), sublaminar cable fixation into C3 laminae (using Nesplon tapes), and insertion of occipital screw. Posterior bone graft from C0 to C3 was performed after instrumentation. Neurological deficits and occipital pain had resolved. The postoperative CT scan (C3 level) shows accurate placement of the pedicle screws, which were inserted into narrow pedicles (Figure 4).

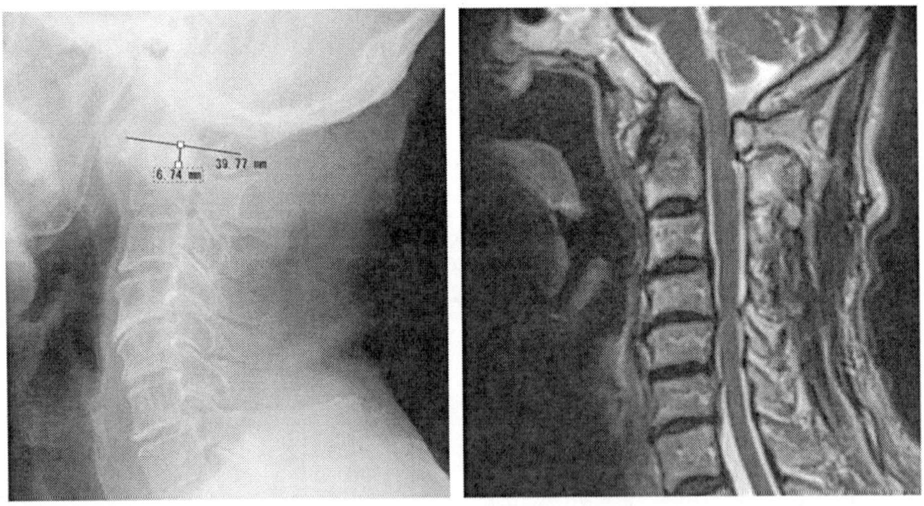

Figure 3. A Preoperative lateral X-ray in a 68-year-old male indicates non-reducible atlanto-axial subluxation and vertical subluxation. B Preoperative sagittal T2-WI MRI shows cord compression due to C1 laminae.

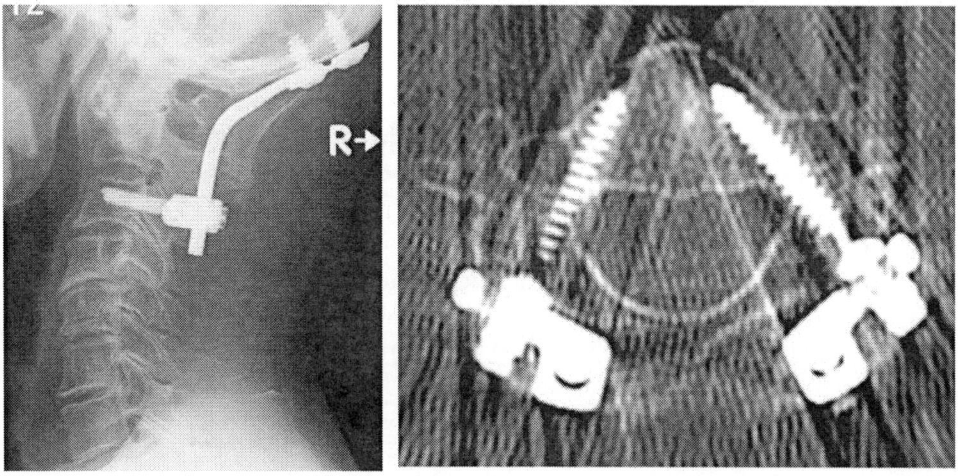

Figure 4. A C1 laminectomy and C0-3 posterior fusion with cervical pedicle screw was performed. B The C3 pedicle screw was accurately positioned

Discussion

Cervical reconstruction surgery should be considered to maintain the quality of life and daily activities in RA patients with severe cervical involvements. A recent study indicated that the natural course of RA patients with myelopathy managed by conservative treatments is poor [24]. In their study, all patients did not recover and were bedridden. Furthermore, all patients had died within 3 years [24]. Casey [25] reported that no benefit was obtained except pain relief by surgical treatment of patients of Ranawat's class 3B. In contrast, the current study showed the potential importance of surgery for class 3B patients, which provided excellent clinical results.

One of the main goals of cervical reconstruction surgery in RA patients is to eliminate instability by achieving immediate and long-term stability. Pedicle screw fixation and C1/2 transarticular screw fixation are biomechanically superior to other conventional procedures using wiring or clamping [6, 7, 22, 26]. Furthermore, pedicle screw fixation is a useful technique because laminectomy or laminoplasty can be performed simultaneously. Conventional screw insertion techniques for both C1/2 screw and pedicle screw placement in the subaxial cervical spine rely on anatomical landmarks and intraoperative fluoroscopy. However, in RA patients, several specific illness-related problems of the cervical spine make surgical treatment extremely difficult. The use of corticosteroid medication for several years and immobilization of the spine caused by multiple musculoskeletal deformities and dysfunctions lead to considerable osteoporosis. Moreover, due to erosion of the anatomical structures, bony landmarks are not always reliable. Especially when the vertebral artery runs an abnormal course, screw placement has a potential risk of neurovascular injury, and vertebral artery injury on the dominant side can cause cerebellar infarction and possibly fetal sequelae [27-29]. Moreover, due to severe spinal deformity and small anatomical size of the vertebra (the lateral mass and pedicle) in the most RA cervical lesions, screw placement procedures are highly technically demanding and pose the potential risk of neurovascular injuries even though intraoperative fluoroscopy is used.

The current study clearly shows from clinical results that computer-assisted screw insertion in the rheumatoid cervical spine enables a significant reduction in the screw malplacement rates (1/40; 2.5%) as compared to conventional insertion techniques, using image intensifier (5.3%; Abumi K et al. [26]). All procedures performed at this facility were performed using a navigation system, therefore no control data is available. Borm et al. [30] reported that transarticular C1–C2 screw fixation was performed in 14 cases using computer navigation (STN 4.0; Zeiss Company, Oberkochen Germany). In this study, there was one medial perforation of a C2 pedicle wall and one malposition of the screw in C2 without reaching the lateral mass of C1 (2/28; 7.1%). In contrast, there were no malpositions of the transarticular C1–C2 screw fixation among our cases.

Regarding C1-2 transarticular screw fixation, it is very easy to navigate at C2 levels using image-guidance systems. However, C1 is easily moved in the prone position even if a Halo-vest apparatus is adapted for patients with atlantoaxial subluxation. In such a case, it is difficult to navigate the screw in the lateral mass of the atlas, and a two-dimensional image intensifier during surgery should be employed. However, this type of image intensifier was not used in pedicle screw insertion in this study. When pedicle perforation was suspected, it was investigated on X-ray image using a marker. Importantly, although the risk of screw perforation can be reduced using a navigation system, its incidence does not disappear completely. Due to the fragile bone quality of the RA cervical spine, care must be taken during rod or plate application procedures and reduction maneuvers which may cause cut-out and displacement of the screw from its original position. To prevent these injuries, preoperative evaluation of the vertebral artery and planning of screw insertion are indispensable. Generally, insertion of screws into the pedicle of less than 3.5 mm in diameter should be avoided even with navigation assistance.

Preoperative vertebral artery evaluation by MR angiography revealed unilateral stenosis or occlusion in 23.8% of patients, all of whom were complicated with VS. Abnormality of vertebral artery is highly likely in RA patients because of cervical deformity. Tumialan et al. [31] reported cerebral and cerebellar infarction in rheumatoid cervical spine patients caused by vertebral artery injury, observed during anterior corpectomy. In consideration of that report, in case of vertebral artery occlusion or stenosis, no pedicle screws were used on the artery-dominant side to avoid vertebrobasilar ischaemia and concurrent stroke if pedicle diameter was narrow. This approach shows significant benefits of preoperative planning using the navigation system. The accuracy of a computer-assisted image-guidance system for correct pedicle screw fixation of the cervical spine has been confirmed in laboratory tests [17], but its clinical results in RA patients have not been clarified. Although the current study was not large in number of patients, the results of surgery under the image-guidance system were encouraging. Use of this system in cervical instrumentation surgery for RA patients can aid in reducing the risk of screw misplacement.

Conclusion

In this study, the authors demonstrated that image guidance systems can be applied safely to the cervical lesions caused by RA. Image-guidance systems are useful tools in preoperative planning and in transpedicular screw placement in the cervical spine of RA patients. However, incidence of screw perforation does not disappear completely. Due to the fragile bone quality of RA cervical spine, care must be taken during rod or plate application procedures and reduction maneuvers. Cervical reconstruction of RA cervical spine using Magerl screw and/or pedicle screw showed relatively stable long-term outcome.

References

[1] Clark, C. R. (1994). Rheumatoid involvement of the cervical spine. An overview. *Spine*, *19*, 2257-2258.

[2] Sharp, J., Purser, D. W. & Lawrence, J. S. (1958). Rheumatoid arthritis of the cervical spine in the adult. *Ann Rheum Dis.*, *17*, 303-313.

[3] Ranawat, C. S., O'Leary, P. & Pellici, P. (1979) Cervical spine fusion in rheumatoid arthritis. *J Bone Joint Surg*, *61A*, 1003-1010.

[4] Santavirta, S., Konttinen, Y., Laasonen, E., Honkanen, V., Antti- Poika, I. & Kauppi, M. (1991). Ten-year results of operations for rheumatoid cervical spine disorders. *J Bone Joint Surg.*, *73B*, 116-120.

[5] Sumi, M., Kataoka, O., Ikeda, M., Sawamura, S., Uno, K. & Siba, R. (1997). Atlantoaxial dislocation: a follow-up study of surgical results. *Spine*, *22*, 759-764.

[6] Grob, D., Crisco, J. J. 3rd, Panjabi, M. M., Wang, P. & Dvorak, J. (1992). Biomechanical evaluation of four different posterior atrantoaxial fixation techniques. *Spine*, *17*, 480-490.

[7] Kotani, Y., Cunningham, B. W., Abumi, K. & McAfee, P. C. (1994). Biomechanical analysis of cervical stabilization systems: an assessment of transpedicular screw fixation in the cervical spine. *Spine*, *17*, 2529-2539.

[8] Jones, E. L., Heller, J. G., Silcox, D. H. & Hutton, W. C. (1997). Cervical pedicle screws versus lateral mass screws. Anatomic feasibility and biomechanical comparison. *Spine*, *22*, 977-982.

[9] Fuji, T., Oda, T., Kato, Y., Fujita, S. & Tanaka, M. (2000). Accuracy of atlantoaxial transarticular screw insertion. *Spine*, *25*, 1760-1764.

[10] Madawi, A. A., Casey, A. T., Solanki, G. A., Tuite, G., Veres, R. & Crockard, H. A. (1997). Radiological and anatomical evaluation of the atrantoaxial transarticular screw fixation technique. *J Neurosurg*, *86*, 961-968.

[11] Wright, N. M. & Lauryssen, C. (1998). Vertebral artery injury in C1-2 transarticular screw fixation: results of a survey of the AANS/CNS Association of Neurological Surgeon/Congress of Neurological Surgeons. *J Neurosurg*, *88*, 634-640.

[12] Golfinos, J. G., Fitzpatrick, B. C., Smith, L. R. & Spetzler, R. F. (1995). Clinical use of a flameless stereotactic arm: results of 325 cases. *J Neurosurg*, *83*, 197-205.

[13] Amiot, L. P., Labelle, H., DeGuise, J. A., Sati, M., Brodeur, P. & Rivard, C. H. (1995). Computer-assist pedicle screw fixation. A feasibility study. *Spine*, *20*, 1208-1212.

[14] Nolte, L. P., Zamorano, L. J., Jiang, Z., Wang, Q., Langlotz, F. & Berlemann, U. (1995). Image-guided insertion of transpedicular screws. A laboratory set-up. *Spine, 20*, 497-500.

[15] Laine, T., Lund, T., Ylikoski, M., Lohikoski, J. & Schlenzka, D. (2000). Accuracy of pedicle screw insertion with and without computer assistance: a randomized controlled clinical study in 100 consecutive patients. *Eur Spine J, 9*, 234-240.

[16] Kamimura, M., Ebara, S., Itoh, H., Tateiwa, Y., Kinoshita, T. & Takaoka, K. (1999). Accurate pedicle screw insertion under control using a computer-assisted image guiding system: laboratory test and clinical study. *J Orthop Sci., 4*, 197-206.

[17] Kamimura, M., Ebara, S., Itoh, H., Tateiwa, Y., Kinoshita, T. & Takaoka, K. (2000). Safe and accurate cervical pedicle screw insertion guided by a computer assisted image-guidance system. *J Spinal Disord, 13*, 218-225.

[18] Takahashi, J., Shono, Y., Nakamura, I., Hirabayashi, H., Kamimura, M., Ebara, S. & Kato, H. (2007). Computer-assisted screw insertion for cervical disorders in rheumatoid arthritis. *Eur Spine J*, 16, 485-494.

[19] Takahashi, J., Hirabayashi, H., Hashidate, H., Ogihara, N. & Kato, H. Accuracy of Multilevel Registration in Image-guided Pedicle Screw Insertion for Adolescent Idiopathic Scoliosis. (2010). *Spine, 35*, 347-352.

[20] Uehara, M., Takahashi, J., Hirabayashi, H., Hashidate, H., Ogihara, N., Mukaiyama, K., Ikegami, S. & Kato, H. (2010). Perforation rates of cervical pedicle screw insertion by disease and vertebral level. (2010). *The Open Orthopaedic Journal, 4*, 142-6.

[21] Ogihara, N., Takahashi, J., Hirabayashi, H., Hashidate, H. & Kato H. Long -term Results of Computer-assisted Posterior Occipito-cervical Reconstruction. *World Neurosurgery* (in press)

[22] Magerl, F. & Seemann, P. S. (1987). Stable posterior fusion of the atlas and axis by transarticular screw fixation. In: P. Kehr, & A. Weidner, (eds) *Cervical spine I*. Springer, Berlin Heidelberg New York, 322-327.

[23] Ranawat, C. S., O'Leary, P., Pellici. P., Tsairis, P., Marchisello, P. & Dorr, L. (1979). Cervical spine fusion in rheumatoid arthritis. *J Bone Joint Surg Am., 61*, 1003-10.

[24] Sunahara, N., Matsunaga, S., Mori, T., Ijiri, K. & Sakou, T. (1997). Clinical course of conservatively managed rheumatoid arthritis patients with myelopathy. *Spine, 22*, 2603-2608.

[25] Casey, A. T. H., Crockard, H. A., Bland, J. M., Stevens, J., Moskovich, R. & Ransford, A. O. (1996). Surgery on the rheumatoid cervical spine for the non-ambulant myelopathic patients-too much, too late? *Lancet, 347*, 1004-1007.

[26] Abumi, K., Kaneda, K., Shono, Y. & Fujiya, M. (1999). One-stage posterior decompression and reconstruction of the cervical spine by using pedicle screw fixation systems. *J Neurosurg (Spine 1), 90*, 19-26.

[27] Abumi, K., Shono, Y., Ito, M., Taneichi, H., Kotani, Y. & Kaneda K. (2000). Complications of pedicle screw fixation in reconstructive surgery of the cervical spine. *Spine, 25*, 962-969.

[28] Shintani, A. & Zervas, N. T. (1972). Consequence of ligation of the vertebral artery. *J Neurosurg, 36*, 447-450.

[29] Smith, M. D., Emery, S. E., Dudley, A., Murray, K. J. & Leventhal, M. (1993), Vertebral artery injury during anterior decompression of the cervical spine. A retrospective review of ten patients. *J Bone Joint Surg, 75B*, 410-415.

[30] Borm, W., Konig, R. W., Albrecht, A., Richter, H. P. & Kast, E. (2004). Percutaneous transarticular atlantaxial screw fixation using a cannulated screw system and image guidance. *Minim Invasive Neurosurg*, *47*, 111-114.

[31] Tumialan, L. M., Wippold, F. J. & 2nd, Morgan, R. A. (2004). Tortuous vertebral artery injury complicating anterior cervical spinal fusion in a symptomatic rheumatoid cervical spine. *Spine*, *29*, E343-E348.

In: Rheumatoid Arthritis: Prevalence, Risk...
Editor: Michael H. Madsen
ISBN: 978-1-61761-931-1

Chapter 6

The Impact of Rheumatic Arthritis on Sexual Function

Antonio G Tristano[*]
Rheumatology Department, Centro Médico Docente La Trinidad,
Caracas, Venezuela, and Centro Médico Carpetana, Madrid, Spain

Introduction

Rheumatoid arthritis (RA) is a chronic inflammatory autoimmune disease characterized by progressive joint destruction resulting from chronic synovial inflammation. It leads to various degrees of disability, and ultimately has a profound impact on the social, economic, psychological, and sexual aspects of the patient's life. The percentage of arthritic patients who experience sexual problems ranged in various studies from 31 to 76%. The reasons for disturbing sexual functioning are multifactorial and comprise disease-related factors as well as therapy. It can occur before, during and after sexual activities, and can affect sexual health in different perspectives.

Sexuality is a complex aspect of the human being's life and is more than of only the sexual act. Normal sexual functioning consists of sexual activity with transition through the phases from arousal to relaxation with no problems, and with a feeling of pleasure, fulfillment and satisfaction. Rheumatic diseases may affect all aspects of life including sexual functioning.

The treatment of sexual dysfunction will depend on the specific patient's symptoms, however, there are some general recommendations including: exploring different positions, using analgesics drug, heat and muscle relaxants before sexual activity and exploring alternative methods of sexual expression.

There are not enough studies comparing sexual functioning between RA patients and healthy controls. However, there is a tendency to find more sexual functioning problems in

[*] Corresponding author: E-mail: antoniotristano@yahoo.com , 5150 NW 99th Ave. Miami FL 33178

patients with RA. These patients could experience sexual disability and diminish sexual drive, with pain and depression being the most common symptoms. This chapter is about the impact of RA on sexual functioning.

The Sexual Function in RA Patients

Sexual functioning is a neglected area of quality of life in patients with RA that is not routinely addressed by physicians or health professionals. Sexual functioning is also not a part of questionnaires frequently used to assess physical function or quality of life. In a recent survey of ten rheumatologists, only 12% of patients seen in their practice were screened for sexual activity. The reasons given by rheumatologists were time constraints, discomfort with the subject, and ambivalence whether such a screening is in their domain or not [1].

The sexual problems in RA could be attributed to physical and psychological variables. Physical variables include difficulties in performing sexual intercourse (sexual disability), while psychological variables include depression, altered body image, worries about partner interest, and diminished sexual drive reflected in both diminished desire and satisfaction. [2-7}]. Difficulty in assuming certain positions when hip or knee movements are limited, dyspareunia due to vaginal dryness in secondary Sjogren's syndrome, and joint pain and fatigue during the intercourse are the principals manifestations of sexual disability, the later is experienced by 50-61% of RA patients [4,8,9].

The majority of patients with RA are female, and there are differences in sexual health between women and men with RA [10]. It has been showed that women with RA have fewer sexual fantasies and masturbate less than controls, and during intercourse, pain is the dominant problem, as well as limited joint mobility [8,11], but there were not differences in satisfaction.

On the other hand, in a study of male adolescents and adults with juvenile idiopathic arthritis (JIA) masturbation and intercourse were practiced equally between patients and controls, although joint pain during intercourse was significantly more frequent among patients. Moreover, although some patients experienced joint pain associated with greater functional disability as indicated by higher HAQ scores, overall sexual pleasure and satisfaction were preserved [12. In contrast, van Berlo et al [11] found that adult males with RA felt less sexual desire than controls (Healthy volunteers), however, patients do not differ from controls regarding sexual satisfaction.

Packham et al [13], in a study of 246 adult's patients with long-standing JIA, found that 50% of them had a detrimental effect on body image but only 28.2% of the patients experienced problems with their relationships. The percentage of patients who were sexually active or had had previous sexual experience was 83.3%; 58.3% of these had disease-related sexual problems. Fewer patients (42.8%) were in stable relationships than their siblings (55.3%). Hill et al [14], studied fifty-eight adults with an average of 14.5 years after the diagnosis of juvenile rheumatoid arthritis. They found that two thirds had mild to moderate disease, good sexual adjustment and "normal" educational achievement, employment history and lifestyle. One third had severe disease, often with progressive disability; this did not prevent sexual activity but caused some limitations.

A possible explication of those differences between young and adult patients could be by the fact that JIA manifests in childhood before the establishment of definite links, relationships, and complete growth. Thus, these limited children are able and have the opportunity and possibility to learn and build up new strategies and developmental mechanisms, such as alternative movements, gestures, and sexual positions, indicating better adaptive skills related to his new reality and life aspects, including sexual functioning [12].

In contrast with this theory, Foster et al [15], evaluated quality of life (QOL) in adults with JIA, and they found that the SF-36 scores for bodily pain, general health, physical functioning, vitality, emotion, and social isolation were significantly worse in patients compared with controls, and this trend increased with increasing age of the patients and disease duration. The SF-36 mental summation scores of patients were low compared with those of controls, for all subtypes of JIA, and this finding was independent of the degree of functional disability. Furthermore, despite excellent educational attainment, there was a high rate of unemployment among patients.

Another important question is whether or not there is any difference between patients with early RA compared with RA patients with long-standing disease. Karlsson et al [16], found that patients with early RA were less satisfied with life as a whole at disease onset compared to patients with long standing disease. Patients with early RA also reported low levels of satisfaction with self-care activities, work and sexual life. The women reported themselves more satisfied than men. Notably, women report themselves less satisfied with sexual life after two years of disease duration. Women with long-standing disease report even lower levels of satisfaction. No correlation was found between disease activity variables and satisfaction with life as a whole. There were, however, positive correlations between disease activity and both satisfaction with partnership and with family life after two years. In patients with early RA compared with those who have chronic RA, the early intervention in addition to the modern early pharmacological treatment practiced today will hopefully lead to a higher degree of life satisfaction.

On the other hand, it is recognized that the androgenic status could be in relation with sexual function. However, hypogonadism or testicular dysfunctions do not necessarily reduce sexual activity. In a study by Gordon et al [17], showed that RA can cause hypogonadism with sexual dysfunction such as impotence and decreased libido.

Impact of Physical and Psychological Variables in Sexual Function in RA Patients

The two mainly sexual problems experienced in RA patients are: difficulties in performing sexual intercourse (sexual disability) and diminished sexual drive reflected in both diminished desire and satisfaction.

Hill et al [18], found that 56% of RA patients reported that arthritis placed limitations on sexual intercourse mainly due to fatigue and pain. It has been showed that when the hip joint are severely affected, total hip replacement improves sexual disability to predisease levels in 50% of sexually active patients with RA [19]. On the other hand, diminished sexual drive is manifested by a decrease in desire in 50–60% of RA patients, reduced frequency of intercourse in up to 73% of patients, increase in aversion to sexual interactions, and diminished sexual satisfaction over time compared to predisease levels [4,8,9].

Elst et al [20], showed that 50% of patients with RA lost sexual interest during the course of their disease and 60% were dissatisfied with quality of their sex life. However, Ostensen et al [21], in a study of patients with history of juvenile chronic arthritis (JCA) showed that in the younger age group and patients with inactive or less active disease, sexual activity and frequency of intercourse was not different from healthy, age-matched controls. Beside, female patients who shared characteristics of marital status with their healthy counterparts showed a similar attitude to sexual activity.

Other studies attributed sexual problems in RA to psychological variables such as depression, altered body image, and worries about partner interest [2-7].

Beside, it has been found that in healthy females, anxiety is associated with reduced frequency of intercourse, whereas depression is an important factor in both loss of libido and loss of sexual satisfaction [6,7].

Kraaimaat et al [22] found that physical disability, pain, and depression all contribute to the intrusiveness of RA on sexuality. Gutweniger et al [23] found that morning stiffness in female RA patients plays an important role in their feelings of being a handicap. Female RA patients with a high degree of morning stiffness also had significantly more worries about body image and experienced more sexual dissatisfaction than females with lower degrees of morning stiffness.

Recently, Abdel-Nasser et al [24], studied 52 females patients with RA They found that 32 patients had difficulties in sexual performance including 9 patients who were totally unable to engage in sexual intercourse because of arthritis. Sexual desire or satisfaction were diminished in 24 patients and completely lost in 24 patients. More than 60% of female RA patients experienced variable degrees of sexual disability and diminished sexual desire and satisfaction. Difficulties in sexual performance were related more to overall disability and hip involvement, while diminished desire and satisfaction were influenced more by perceived pain, age, and depression. They also found that 27% of their patients had genital tract abnormalities that could influence sexual performance. However, these abnormalities can be easily controlled by prompt gynecological referral.

In another recent study, van Berlo et al [11] found that male patients felt less sexual desire, and female patients masturbated and fantasized less than controls. Differences in satisfaction were not found. Male and female patients did not experience more sexual problems than controls. Up to 41% of the men, and up to 51% of the women have troubles with several joints during sexual activities. Medications influencing ejaculation in men correlated with distress with orgasm.

Impact of RA in Couple's Relationship

Majerovitz et al [25], when examined the relationship between functional disability and sexual satisfaction for both rheumatic disease patients and their spouses and compared their levels of sexual satisfaction to those of healthy comparison couples, they found that rheumatic disease and comparison couples did not differ in sexual dissatisfaction. However, greater functional disability was related to greater sexual dissatisfaction for patients and spouses.

Bermas et al [26)], in a cross-sectional survey of 79 persons with RA and 78 spouses correlated their marital satisfaction. They found that patients and spouses were generally satisfied with their marriages. Besides, it was showed that lower marital satisfaction in patients was associated with higher education level, patient's greater use of escape into fantasy, patient's greater use of finding blame, and spouse's higher use of escape into fantasy. Spouses less satisfied with their marriages were more likely to use passive acceptance and less likely to find blame. Female spouses were less likely to be satisfied in their marriages than male spouses. They concluded that certain passive coping styles, more highly educated patients and female spouses are associated with lower marital satisfaction in persons with RA and their spouses.

Kraaimaat et al [22], studied whether physical disability, pain, depressive mood, and criticism by the spouse are differentially related to intrusiveness of RA on sexuality in male and female patients. They assessed physical and psychological aspects of health in 102 male and 118 female RA patients who were living with a spouse. They found that physical disability, pain, and, to a lesser extent, depression were found to contribute to intrusiveness of RA on sexuality. However, female patients, compared with male patients, appeared to have lower levels of mobility and self-care. They suggested that differences in sexual motivation between men and women might have been influential in the absence of gender differences in intrusiveness.

Treatment Recommendations

One of the most important issues about the treatment of sexual dysfunction associated to RA is the fact that neither the sexual functioning is routinely addressed by physicians or health professionals, nor it is part of frequently used questionnaires to assess physical function or quality of life. For example, in Europe, especially UK health professionals should monitor the sexual activity of RA patients; however, a recent study showed that 66% of RA patients were never asked about the impact of RA on their sexual lives [18]. The common problem is communication, so an open communication including inquiry about sexuality into the routine care is the first step to improve the situation. To allow the patients to present problems and concerns without embarrassment is also important. After an open communication is achieved, the treatment will depend on the specific patient's symptoms (Table 1). However, there are some general recommendations including: discussion of the problems with the partner, principally about the partner's fear in causing pain or distress during sexual intercourse, exploring different positions, using analgesics drug, heat, and muscle relaxants before, sexual activity in order to decrease pain, and exploring alternative methods of sexual expression [27,28].

Table 1. Factors Associated To Sexual Dysfunction In Rheumatoid Arthritis And Recommendations For Specific Symptoms

Sexual dysfunction	Factors implicated	Recommendations
Sexual disability	Limited mobility	Change position
	Pain, fatigue	Analgesic, heat, and muscle
	Morning stiffness	Relaxation before activity, Surgery.
Dyspareunia	Vaginal dryness	Vaginal lubrication, estrogen cream.
Diminished desire and Satisfaction	Anxiety, depression Altered body image	Counseling, antidepresive drugs[a]
Impotence	Hormonal imbalance	Sidenafil, sex therapy.

a Could decrease libido (Modificated from Tristano 2009)

References

[1] Britto, MT; Rosenthal, SL; Taylor, J; Passo, MH. Improving rheumatologists' screening for alcohol use and sexual activity. *Arch Pediatr Adolesc Med*, 2000, 154(5), 478-483.

[2] Ehrlich, GE. Social, economic, psychologic, and sexual outcomes in rheumatoid arthritis. *Am J Med*, 1983, 75, 27-34.

[3] Blake, DJ; Maisiak, R; Koplan, A; eAlarcón, GS; Brown, S. Sexual dysfunction among patients with arthritis. *Clin Rheumatol*, 1988, 7, 50-60.

[4] Blake, DJ; Maisiak, R; Alarcon, GS; Holley, HL; Brown, S. Sexual quality-of-life of patients with arthritis compared to arthritis-free controls. *J Rheumatol*, 1987, 14(3), 570-576.

[5] van Lankveld, W; Ruiterkamp, G; Naring, G; de Rooji, DJ. Marital and sexual satisfaction in patients with RA and their spouses. *Scand J Rheumatol*, 2004, 33(6), 405-408.

[6] Channon, LD; Ballinger, SE. Some aspects of sexuality and vaginal symptoms during menopause and their relation to anxiety and depression. *Br J Med Psychol*, 1986, 59, 173-180.

[7] Frohlich, P; Meston, C. Sexual functioning and self-reported depressive symptoms among college women. *J Sex Res.*, 2002, 39, 321-325.

[8] Yoshino, S; Uchida, S. Sexual problems of women with rheumatoid arthritis. *Arch Phys Med Rehabil*, 1981, 62(3), 122-123.

[9] Bhadauria, S; Moser, DK; Clements, PJ; Singh, RR; Lachenbruch, PA; Pitkin, RM; Weiner, SR. Genital tract abnormalities and female sexual function impairment in systemic sclerosis. *Am J Obstet Gynecol*, 1995, 172, 580-587.

[10] Areskoug-Josefsson, K; Oberg, U. A literature review of the sexual health of women with rheumatoid arthritis. *Musculoskeletal Care*. 2009, 7(4), 219-26.

[11] van Berlo, WT; van de Wiel, HB; Taal, E; Rasker, JJ; Weijmar Schultz, WC; van Rijswijk, MH. Sexual functioning of people with rheumatoid arthritis: a multicenter study. *Clin Rheumatol*, 2007, 26(1), 30-38.

[12] de Avila Lima Souza, L; Gallinaro, AL; Abdo, CH; Kowalski, SC; Suehiro, RM; da Silva, CA; Goldenstein-Schainberg, C. Effect of musculoskeletal pain on sexuality of male adolescents and adults with juvenile idiopathic arthritis. *J Rheumatol*, 2009, 36(6), 1337-42.

[13] Packham, JC; Hall, MA; Pimm, TJ. Long-term follow-up of 246 adults with juvenile idiopathic arthritis: predictive factors for mood and pain. *Rheumatology (Oxford)*, 2002, 41(12), 1444-9.

[14] Hill, RH; Herstein, A; Walters, K. Juvenile rheumatoid arthritis: follow-up into adulthood-medical, sexual and social status. *Can Med Assoc J*, 1977, 114, 790-794.

[15] Foster, HE; Marshall, N; Myers, A; Dunkley, P; Griffiths, ID. Outcome in adults with juvenile idiopathic arthritis: a quality of life study. *Arthritis Rheum*, 2003, 48(3), 767-75.

[16] Karlsson, B; Berglin, E; Wållberg-Jonsson, S. Life satisfaction in early rheumatoid arthritis: a prospective study. *Scand J Occup Ther.*, 2006, 13(3), 193-199.

[17] Gordon, D; Beastall, GH; Thomson, JA; Sturrock, RD. Androgenic status and sexual function in males with rheumatoid arthritis and ankylosing spondylitis. *QJM*, 1986, 60, 671-679.

[18] Hill, J; Bird, H; Thorpe, R. Effects of rheumatoid arthritis on sexual activity and relationships. *Rheumatology (Oxford)*, 2003, 42(2), 280-286.

[19] Yoshino, S; Fujimori, J; Morishige, T; Uchida, S. Bilateral joint replacement of hip and knee joints in patients with rheumatoid arthritis. *Arch Orthop Trauma Surg.*, 1984, 103(1), 1-4

[20] Elst, R; Sybesma, T; van der Stadt, RJ; Prins, AP; Muller, WH; den Butter, A. Sexual problems in rheumatoid arthritis and ankylosing spondylitis. *Arthritis Rheum*, 1984, 27, 217-220.

[21] Østensen, M; Almberg, K; Koksvik, H. Sex, reproduction, and gynecological disease in young adults with a history of juvenile chronic arthritis. *J Rheumatol*, 2000, 27, 1783-1787.

[22] Kraaimaat, FW; Bakker, AH; Janssen, E; Bijlsma, JW. Intrusiveness of rheumatoid arthritis on sexuality in male and female patients living with a spouse. *Arthritis Care Res.*, 1996, 9, 120-125.

[23] Gutweniger, S; Kopp, M; Mur, E; Gunther, V. Body image of women with rheumatoid arthritis. *Clin Exp Rheumatol*, 1999, 17(4), 413-417.

[24] Abdel-Nasser, AM; Ali, EI. Determinants of sexual disability and dissatisfaction in female patients with rheumatoid arthritis. *Clin Rheumatol*, 2006, 25(6), 822-30.

[25] Majerovitz, SD; Revenson, TA. Sexuality and rheumatic disease: the significance of gender. *Arthritis Care Res.*, 1994, 7(1), 29-34.

[26] Bermas, BL; Tucker, JS; Winkelman, DK; Katz, JN. Marital satisfaction in couples with rheumatoid arthritis. *Arthritis Care Res.*, 2000, 13(3), 149-55.

[27] Panush, RS; Mihailescu, GD; Gornisiewicz, MT; Sutaria, SH; Wallace, DJ. Sex and arthritis. *Bull Rheum Dis.*, 2000, 49(7), 1-4.

[28] Tristano, AG. Tyrosine kinases as targets in rheumatoid arthritis. *Int Immunopharmacol.*, 2009, 9(1), 1-9.

In: Rheumatoid Arthritis: Prevalence, Risk...
Editor: Michael H. Madsen
ISBN: 978-1-61761-931-1

Chapter 7

Role of T Cells in Human Osteoclastogenesis - Bone Destruction of Rheumatoid Arthritis via Cytokines from T Cells

Shigeru Kotake*, Yuki Nanke, Toru Yago, Takefumi Furuya, Manabu Kawamoto, Naomi Ichikawa, Tsuyoshi Kobashigawa and Naoyuki Kamatani
Institute of Rheumatology, Tokyo Women's Medical University,
Tokyo, Japan

Abstract

Activated human T cells produce receptor activator NF-κB ligand (RANKL), interleukin-17 (IL-17), and interferon-γ (IFN-γ). All regulate human osteoclastogenesis; RANKL and IL-17 potently induce osteoclastogenesis, while IFN-γ directly inhibits it in vitro. However, we have demonstrated that IFN-γ-producing T cells induce human osteoclastogenesis from monocytes through the expression of RANKL. Strongly supporting our findings, it has been reported that peripheral blood T cells from patients with early rheumatoid arthritis (RA) promote osteoclastogenesis in autologus monocytes through the expression of RANKL, although the T cells express IFN-γ. In addition, it has been reported that IFN-γ has indirect pro-osteoclastogenic properties in vivo; IFN-γ induces bone resorption in three mouse models of osteoporosis under conditions of estrogen deficiency, infection, and inflammation. On the other hand, the expression or function of some cytokines shows differences between humans and mice in bone cell biology. In the current article, we review recent findings on the role of T cells in human

*Correspondence concerning this article should be addressed to: Dr. Shigeru Kotake, Institute of Rheumatology, Tokyo Women's Medical University, 10-22 Kawada-cho, Shinjuku, Tokyo 162-0054 Japan. Tel: 81-3-5269-1725; Fax: 81-3-5269-1726; e-mail: skotake@ior.twmu.ac.jp.

osteoclastogenesis and bone destruction of rheumatoid arthritis (RA), including the effects of dexamethasone and tacrolimus on the function of T cells.

Keywords: dexamethasone, interferon-γ (IFN-γ), interleukin-17 (IL-17), IL-23, rheumatoid arthritis (RA), osteoclast, osteoprogeterin (OPG), receptor activator of NF-κB ligand (RANKL), single nucleotide polymorphism (SNP), tacrolimus (FK506).

Introduction

Since 1990, we have investigated human osteoclastogenesis in the pathogenesis of rheumatoid arthritis (RA) by three hypotheses: 1)to investigate the pathogenesis of RA, it is important to study osteoclastogenesis using human rather than mouse cells; 2)osteoclastogenesis in RA is regulated by a mechanism independent of inflammation; and 3) activated human T cells regulate human osteoclastogenesis.

To investigate the pathogenesis of RA, it is critical to investigate osteoclastogenesis using human cells. In bone cell biology, some cytokines show different functions between humans and mice. For example, macrophage-colony stimulating factor (M-CSF) induces colony formation from mouse cells. In human cells, however, M-CSF induces the differentiation of progenitor cells of monocytes rather than colony formation in human cells, although M-CSF is reported to induce colony formation of human macrophages [1]. On the other hand, some cytokines show different expressions between humans and mice; it is reported that the expression of membrane-bound receptor activator NF-κB ligand (RANKL) is limited in human T cells compared with mouse T cells [2]. Moreover, the mouse CD4+CD25+ regulatory subset is isolated from all CD25+ T cells regardless of their level of CD25 expression; however, when similar criteria are followed to isolate these cells from human blood, CD25+ cells (high and low together) did not exhibit an anergic phenotype or significant suppressive function. In humans, CD4+CD25^{hi} exhibit all properties of regulatory T cells [3,4]. In addition, recently it has been reported that a major difference between humans and mice in immunology is the presence of CD4+T cells producing IL-17, Th17 cells, in healthy peripheral blood of humans, but not mice [5]. Thus, in the study of human diseases, it is essential to investigate human osteoclastogenesis using human cells.

Osteoclastogenesis in RA is regulated by a mechanism, at least in part, independent of inflammation. Osteoclastogenesis dependent on and independent of inflammation has been reported in the pathogenesis of RA since RANKL was cloned as an 'osteoclast differentiation factor (ODF)' in 1997. We recently reported that the amount of T cells expressing both interferon-γ (IFN-γ and RANKL in peripheral blood of patients with RA does not correlate with the serum level of C-reactive protein [6]. On the other hand, it has been reported that mature osteoclasts are inactivated by selectively inhibiting cathepsin K, carbonic anhydrase II or vacuolar-H(+) ATPase, which are essential in bone resorption by osteocalsts. In addition, more recently, Geusens et al. showed that, in joint destruction of patients with early active RA, the effects of inflammation (time-averaged ESR) and osteoclast differentiation/activity (circulating OPG:RANKL ratio) are statistically partly independent and may be superimposed [7]. Thus, nowadays it is possible to regulate bone resorption in RA by a mechanism separate from inflammation.

Activated human T cells regulate human osteoclastogenesis, producing RANKL, interleukin-17 (IL-17), or IFN-γ, all of which regulate human osteoclastogenesis. In addition, it has been demonstrated that these cytokines play a critical role in human osteoclastogenesis *in vitro* as well as bone resorption in patients with rheumatoid arthritis (RA). In the current article, we review recent findings on the role of T cells in human osteoclastogenesis and bone destruction of RA.

1. Osteoclasts

Osteoclasts are unique multinucleated cells whose function is specialized to resorb calcified tissues (Figure 1) [6]. On the surface of bone, osteoclasts develop a specialized adhesion structure, 'podosome', which subsequently undergoes reorganization into sealing zones [8]. These ring-like adhesion structures seal osteoclasts to the surface of bone. In the sealed resorption lacuna, localized acidification is driven by carbonic anhydrase II and vacuolar H(+)-ATPase in osteoclasts; carbonic anhydrase II produces protons and vacuolar H(+)-ATPase transfers them into the lacuna. In acidified lacuna, cathepsin-K and matrix metalloproteinase-9 (MMP-9) are released from osteoclasts to degrade calcified tissues [9].

The cooperation of osteoclasts and osteoblasts is critical to maintain skeletal integrity in normal bone. After bone resorption by osteoclasts on normal bone tissues, osteoblasts subsequently rebuild bone in the lacunae resorbed by osteoclasts; this mechanism is called 'bone remodeling'. When the activity or number of osteoclasts is elevated compared with osteoblasts, the bone become fragile, that is, 'osteoporotic'. In addition, bone remodeling is disrupted in all bone diseases associated with changes in bone mass. Thus, bone remodeling is essential to retain both the structure and strength of normal bone.

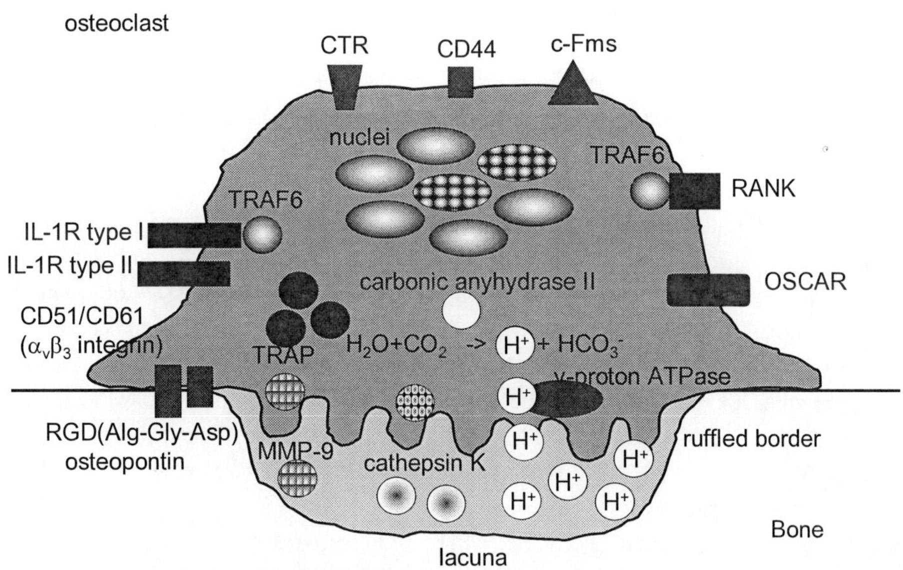

Figure 1. Schematic structure of osteoclasts. CTR, calcitonin receptor; TRAF, TNF receptor-associated factor; TRAP, tartrate-resistant acid phosphatase; MMP, matrix metalloproteinase; OSCAR, osteoclast-associated receptor; c-Fms, M-CSF receptor

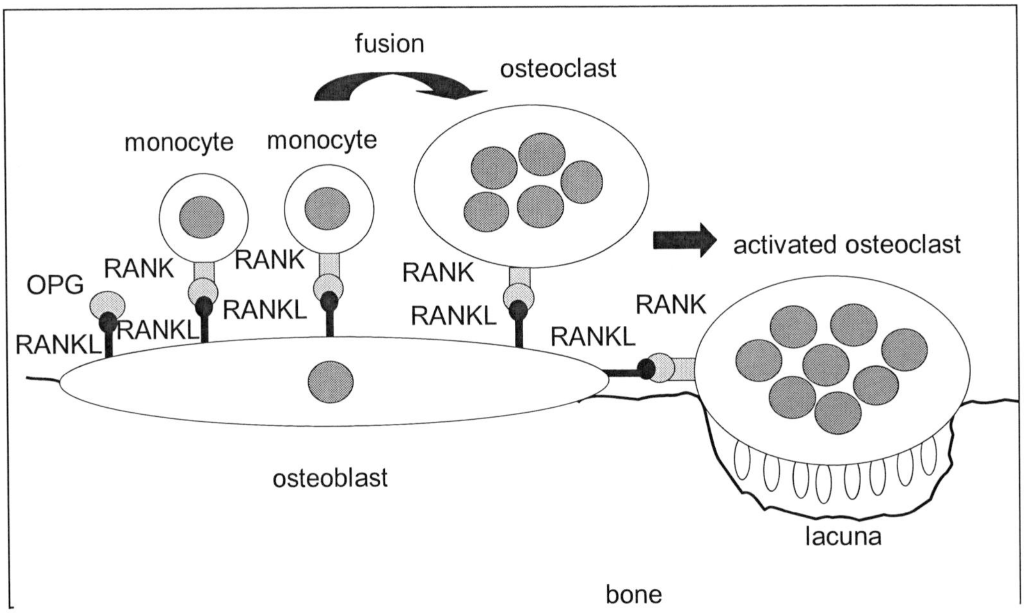

Figure 2. Differentiation and activation of osteoclasts. OPG, osteoprotegerin. A RANK-RANKL system induces both osteoclastogenesis from monocytes and the activation of mature osteoclasts

Osteoclasts also play an important role in the pathogenesis of rheumatoid arthritis (RA). Since 1984, it has been reported that in bone destruction of rheumatoid arthritis (RA), many activated osteoclasts are detected on the surface of eroded bone in the interface with synovial tissues [10]. In addition, we have demonstrated that osteoclasts are detected in synovial tissues as well as eroded bone from patients with RA [11]. In addition, we have reported that the number of precursor cells of osteoclasts increases in bone marrow adjacent to joints with arthritis [12]. Moreover, the amount of cytokines that induce osteoclastogenesis such as IL-1, tumor necrosis factor-α (TNF-α) and IL-6, is elevated in synovial tissues of patients with RA, while the amount of cytokines that inhibit osteoclastogenesis, such as IL-4 and IL-10, is decreased [12-15]. Thus, patients with RA are likely to suffer from joint destruction as well as systemic osteoporosis, in which the number of osteoclasts increases, suggesting that osteoclasts play a critical role in the pathogenesis of RA.

The origin of osteoclasts was unclarified until the 1980s. In 1988, Takahashi et al. established a culture system using mouse spleen cells and osteoblasts to induce osteoclastogenesis *in vitro*, demonstrating that the origin of osteoclasts is hematopoietic cells [16]. The precursor of osteoclasts was then revealed to be colony-forming unit-macrophage (CFU-M) or CFU-granulocyte/macrophage (CFU-GM) in bone marrow or spleen in mice. In 1990, Udagawa et al. demonstrated that osteoclasts are formed from murine macrophages [17]. From these findings, Suda et al. hypothesized that bone marrow hemopoietic cells differentiate into osteoclasts through the stimulation of 'osteoclast-differentiation factor (ODF)' expressed on osteoblasts [18].

Finally, ODF, now termed RANKL, which induces osteoclastogenesis from monocytes or macrophages, was independently cloned by three groups in 1997 (Figure 1) [19]. RANKL is a member of the TNF superfamily of cytokines. The protein constructs a trimeric complex to bind its receptor, receptor activator NF-κB (RANK) (20). A decoy receptor is also cloned, which is designated as 'osteoprotegerin (OPG)' [19] (Figure 2).

2. T Cells Producing RANKL

RANKL expressed on T cells as well as on osteoblasts induces osteoclastogenesis. Two groups reported using murine cells that T cells directly induce murine osteoclastogenesis through the expression of RANKL from T cells [21,22]. We have also demonstrated using human T cells and monocytes that human T cells induce osteoclastogenesis from peripheral human monocytes through the expression of RANKL on T cells (Figure 3) [23]. We have also demonstrated that CD4+ T cells in synovial tissues from patients with RA express RANKL, and that the ratio of levels of RANKL to those of OPG in synovial fluids is elevated (Figure 7) [23]. Thus, in synovial fluids of patients with RA, monocytes are likely to differentiate into osteoclasts.

Strongly supporting our findings, two groups have recently demonstrated important results. First, Miranda-Carus et al. have reported that peripheral blood T cells from patients with RA promote osteoclastogenesis from autologous monocytes through the expression of RANKL on T cells, although T cells simultaneously produce IFN-γ [24]. Thus, they concluded that T cells are important contributors to the pathogenesis of bone erosion in RA through interaction with monocytes. Second, Geusens et al. have reported that the ratio of circulating OPG to RANKL in early RA predicts later joint destruction, analyzing 92 patients with early active RA for 5 years [7]. Thus, the reports on osteoclastogenesis and bone destruction in RA patients in these groups support our findings.

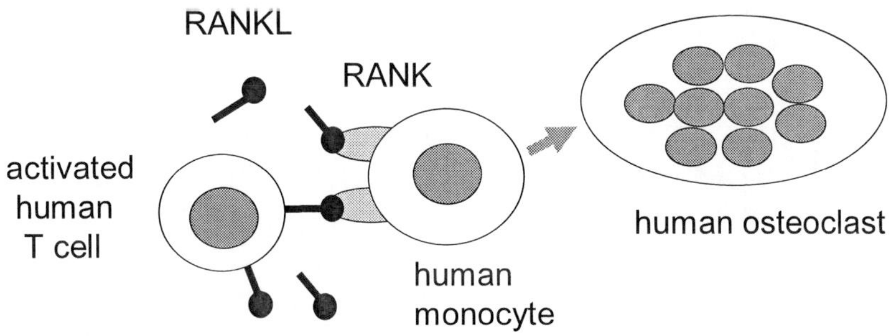

Figure 3. Activated human T cells induce osteoclastogenesis from human monocytes through the expression of RANKL on T cells

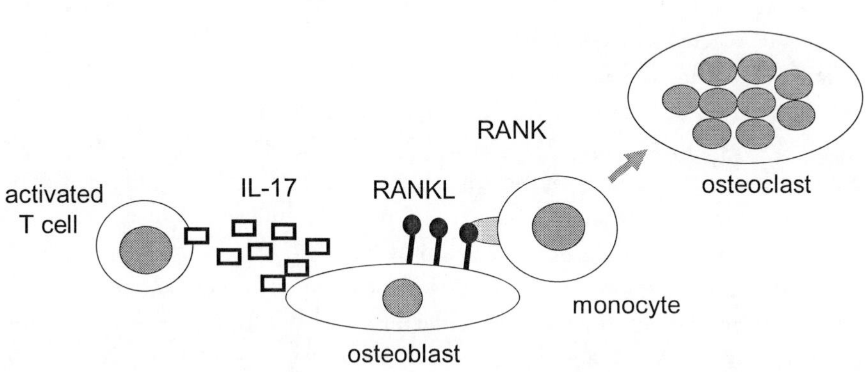

Figure 4. IL-17 from activated T cells induces osteoclastogenesis through the expression of RANKL on osteoblasts

In mature osteoclasts, the function of IL-1 and TNF-α, but not RANKL, shows differences between humans and mice. In both humans and mice, RANKL stimulates bone resorption of mature osteoclasts [9]; however, IL-1 and TNF-α show no significant effects on human mature osteoclasts, which contrasts with the potent ability of both cytokines to stimulate murine mature osteoclasts [9]. On the other hand, we have demonstrated that in both humans and mice, TNF-α directly induces osteoclastogenesis [25]. Thus, the differences in species used in the studies are critical to discuss the function of cytokines.

The pathogenesis of periodontitis is similar to that of RA because both diseases show chronic inflammation. The levels of RANKL are elevated in gingival crevicular fluid of patients with periodontitis [26]. In addition, T cells from patients with periodontitis express RANKL [27]. Interestingly, human T cells expressing RANKL transplanted to NOD/SCID mice show alveolar bone destruction [28]. Recently, it has been reported that the induction of an adaptive immune response to orally colonizing non-pathogenic *Pasteurella pneumotropica* by immunization with phylogenetically closely related bacterium, *Actinobacillus actinomycetemcmitans,* results in T cell-derived RANKL-dependent periodontal bone loss in mice [29]. Thus, T cells expressing RANKL play a critical role in bone destruction of perodontitis.

3. Th17 Cells Producing IL-17

1) IL-17

In 1993, IL-17 was initially identified as a transcript selectively expressed by activated T cells encoding a protein with significant sequence identity (~60%) to the Herpesvirus saimiri protein HVS13 [30]. In 1996, IL-17, which induces IL-6, IL-8, and granulocyte colony-stimulating factor (G-CSF) from stromal cells [31], and IL-1 and TNF-α from macrophages [32], was cloned as a unique interleukin showing a function similar to that of IL-1, although IL-17 is produced by T cells [30]. IL-17 receptor (IL-17R), ubiquitously expressed, was reported to be a unique structure different from any receptors of other interleukins. Recently, however, a bioinformatics study predicted a subdomain in IL-17-family receptors with homology to a Toll/IL-1R (TIR) domain, termed the "SEFIR domain" [33]. More recently, Maitra et al. reported that distinct functional motifs within the IL-17 receptor regulate signal transduction and target gene expression [34].

IL-17and IL-17R have been renamed IL-17A and IL-17RA, respectively; five additional IL-17-like ligands (IL-17B-F) and four additional IL-17R-like receptors (IL-17RB-E) have been identified [35]. Interestingly, Toy et al. reported that the biologic activity of IL-17 is dependent on a heteromeric receptor complex composed of IL-17RA and IL-17RC [36].

In 1999, we first demonstrated that IL-17 potently induces mouse osteoclastogenesis from mouse monocytes through the expression of RANKL of osteoblasts (Figure 4) [32,37]. In addition, we recently reported that IL-17 induces human osteoclastogenesis from human monocytes even in the absence of osteoblastic cells or soluble RANKL through both inductively-expressed TNF-α and constitutively-expressed RANKL on human monocytes [37]. In this osteoclastogenesis, the synergistic effect of TNF-α and RANKL plays an important role; the expressed level of each cytokines is too low to induce osteoclastogenesis in each cytokine alone [37]. This synergism has also been reported by other two groups [38,39]. More recently, it has been reported that peripheral blood T cells from patients with early RA promote osteoclastogenesis in autologous monocytes in the absence of exogenous cytokines or osteoblasts, and that osteoclastogenesis is significantly inhibited by neutralizing monoclonal antibodies to IL-17 [24]. Thus, IL-17 induces osteoclastogenesis from monocytes both in the absence and presence of osteoblasts.

Synovial tissues of patients with RA contain an increased number of T cells; however, using the usual ELISA with standard sensitivity, it was very difficult to detect cytokines derived from T cells, such as IL-2 or IFN-γ, in synovial tissues or synovial fluids. Until 1999, this absence of T cell-derived cytokines was an 'enigma' to be solved in the pathogenesis of RA. We first demonstrated that a sufficient amount of a T cell-derived cytokine, IL-17, is detected in synovial fluids from patients with RA using the usual ELISA (Figure 7) [32]. Lubbers et al. reported that treatment with a neutralizing anti-murine IL-17 antibody after the onset of collagen-induced arthritis (CIA) reduces joint inflammation, cartilage destruction, and bone erosion [41]. We also demonstrated that in rats with CIA, peritoneal injection of anti-IL-17 Ab ameliorates synovitis even after the onset of arthritis [42]. In addition, Nakae et al. also reported that IL-17 play an important role in the pathogenesis of a murine arthritis model [43]. Recently, Sarkar et al. reported that dendritic cells genetically modified to express IL-4 exert a therapeutic effect on CIA by targeting IL-17 [44]. Interestingly, Raza et al. reported that early RA of 3-months duration or less is characterized by a distinct and transient synovial fluid cytokine profile of T cells including IL-17, but not IFN-γ [45]. Thus, IL-17 plays an important role in both human RA and murine arthritis models.

It has been reported that interplay between IL-23 and IL-17 production may be a critical immune pathway using gene-targeted mice lacing IL-23 (p19-/-), which is resistant to CIA induction [46]. We recently demonstrated that IL-23 induces osteoclastogenesis in the culture of human PBMC via the expression of IL-17 from T cells [47]. In addition, peritoneal injection of anti-IL-23 Ab ameliorates synovitis of rats with CIA [47]. Thus, IL-23 may induces osteoclastogenesis upstream of IL-17 in the pathogenesis of RA.

2) Th17

In 2005, a novel subset of helper T cells was demonstrated; Th cells expressing IL-17 distinct from Th1 cells or Th2 cells were designated as Th17, Th_{IL-17}, or inflammatory TH (THi). In 1986, Mosmann et al. demonstrated the dichotomy of helper T cells; Th1 cells producing IFN-γ in cellular immunity and Th2 cells producing IL-4 in humoral immunity [48]. The pathogenesis of many diseases has been divided into two categories; for example, RA is Th1 disease, which we confirmed using peripheral helper T cells from patients with RA treated without any disease-modifying anti-rheumatic drugs (DMARDs) or steroids [6]. On the other hand, bronchial asthma and atopic dermatitis are Th2 diseases. The notion that IL-17-producing T cells may be a distinct T cell lineage emerged from gene-targeted mice models with experimental autoimmune encephalomyelitis (EAE) or CIA [49]. In 2005, two laboratories simultaneously reported IL-17-producing CD4+ T cells (Th17, Th_{IL-17}) as a distinct effector lineage [50,51]. In 2006, it was reported that naïve T cells are primed to Th17 by IL-6 and transforming growing factor (TGF)-β, and that IL-23 stimulates the production of

IL-17 from primed T cells [52-54]. Human Th17 cells have distinct migratory capacity with the expressions of CCR6 and CCR4 together and antigenic specificities for *Candida albicans* [55]. Reports using infectious mouse models have suggested that Th17 cells develop to mediate protection against extracellular bacteria and *Pneumocystis carinii* [56-58]. In addition, it has been reported that Th17 functions as an osteoclastogenic helper T cell subset that links T cell activation and bone destruction [59]. Hirota et al. reported that autoimmune arthritis of SKG mice is highly dependent on the development of Th17 cells [60]. In addition, IL-17 plays an important role in the pathogenesis of periodontitis [61,62]. Thus, Th17 cells may be involved in bone destruction in RA and periodontitis as well as in the pathogenesis of autoimmune disorders of model mouse such as EAE and autoimmune arthritis, whereas Th17 cells develop to mediate protection against fungi and extracellular bacteria.

4. Th1 Cells Producing IFN-γ

IFN-γ produced by Th1 cells plays an important role in the defense of hosts against viruses or intracellular microorganisms. It has been reported that IFN-γ inhibits osteoclastogenesis [63,64]. In 2000, IFN-γ was shown to inhibit mouse osteoclastogenesis through the degradation of TRAF6 *in vitro* and to repress bone resorption in calvariae from prepubertal mice *in vivo* [65].

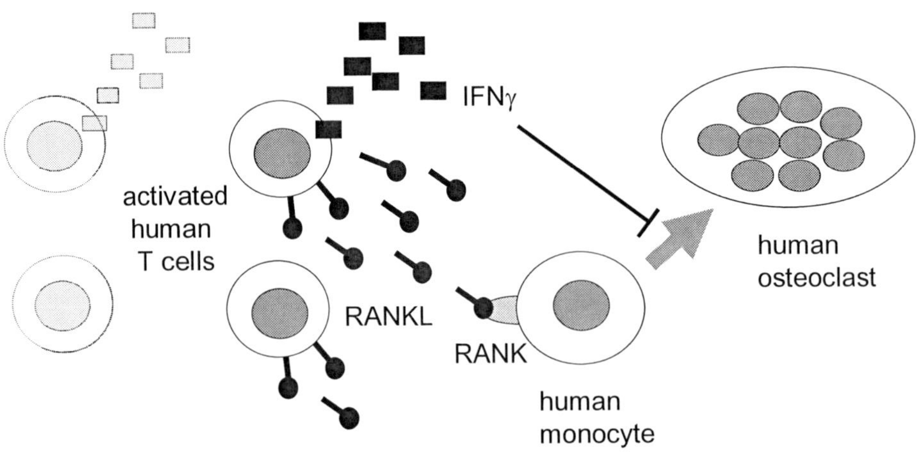

Figure 5. Human activated T cells producing IFN-γ, which simultaneously produce RANKL, induce human osteoclastogenesis from monocytes. IFN-γ from activated T cells inhibits human osteoclastogenesis from monocytes; however, human activated T cells producing IFN-γ, which simultaneously produce RANKL, induce human osteoclastogenesis from monocytes

We have demonstrated that activated human T cells induce human osteoclastogenesis from monocytes though the expression of RANKL [23] as described above (Figure 3). Moreover, we recently reported that human IFN-γ-producing T cells (Th1 cells) induce human osteoclastogenesis from monocytes via the production of RANKL from Th1 cells (Figure 5) and that the number of T cells expressing both IFN-γ and RANKL is elevated in the peripheral blood of patients with RA (Figure 6) [6]. Strongly supporting our findings, it

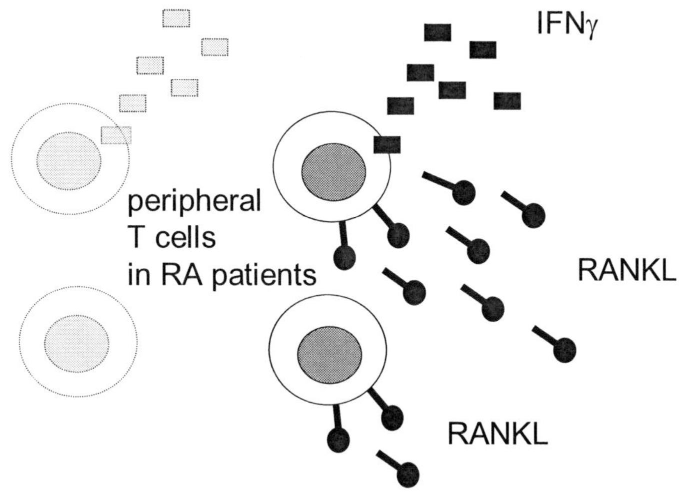

Figure 6. Human helper T cells producing IFN-γ simultaneously produce RANKL in peripheral blood of patients with RA. Theoretically, activated human T cells are divided into 4 types by the production of IFN-γ and RANKL. However, only 2 types, IFN-γ (+), RANKL(+)T cells and IFN-γ (-), RANKL(+)T cells, are detected in peripheral blood of patients with RA

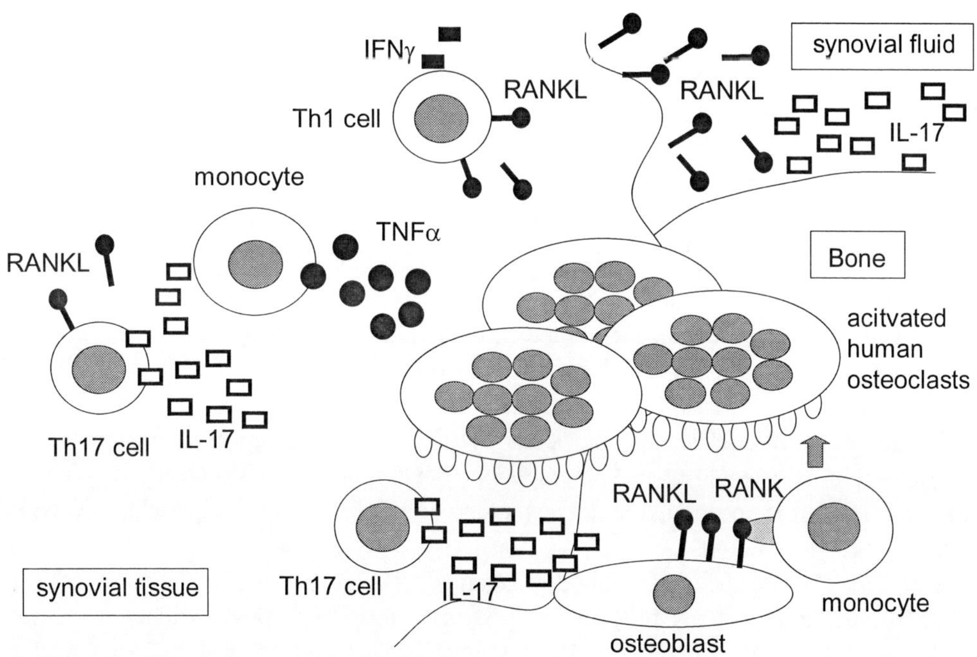

Figure 7. A scheme of the role of T cells in bone resorption in RA. It is speculated that Th17 cells and Th1 cells play an important role in bone resorption in RA through the formation and activation of osteoclasts

has been demonstrated that IFN-γ has indirect pro-osteoclastogenic properties *in vivo*; IFN-γ induces bone resorption in three mouse models with osteoporosis under conditions of estrogen deficiency, infection, and inflammation [66]. In addition, also supporting our findings, Miranda-Carus et al. have reported that peripheral blood T cells from patients with RA promote osteoclastogenesis from autologous monocytes through the expression of RANKL on T cells, although T cells simultaneously produce IFN-γ [24]. Moreover, Stashenko et al. demonstrated using a murine model with periodontitis that Th1 immune response promotes severe bone resorption caused by *Porphyromonas gingivalis* [67]. Thus, IFN-γ or Th1 cells may play a critical role in indirect bone resorption and destruction in a murine model *in vivo* and patients with RA, although IFN-γ directly inhibits murine and human osteoclastogenesis from monocytes *in vitro*.

5. Regulatory T Cells

Regulatory T cells (Tregs) are a subset of CD4+ T cells expressing CD25 with immunosuppressive activity. Recently, it has been reported that Tregs inhibit human osteoclastogenesis from PBMC [68]. This suppression of osteoclastogenesis was blocked by anti-TGF-β antibody or anti-IL-4 antibody, suggesting that TGF-β and IL-4 are key cytokines for the suppressive function of Tregs. On the other hand, it has been reported that TNF downmodulates the function of human CD4+CD25^{hi} Tregs [4]. In fact, CD4+CD25^{hi} Tregs isolated from patients with active RA poorly suppress the proliferation and cytokine secretion of CD4+ effector T cells [4], Thus, the reduced function of Tregs in patients with RA might, at least in part, limit the inhibition of osteoclasts, inducing elevated bone resorption.

6. Cell-Cell Fusion in Osteoclastogenesis

Dendritic cell-specific transmembrane protein (DC-STAMP) is a seven-transmembrane protein originally identified in dendritic cells [69]. Kukita et al. reported that DC-STAMP is essential for the differentiation of osteoclasts, showing that the expression of DC-STAMP is rapidly induced in osteoclast precursor cells by RANKL [70]. Yagi et al. demonstrated that multinucleation of osteoclasts and macrophages is completely abrogated in DC-STAMP -/- mice [71]. Thus, it is speculated that T cells play an important role in inducing DC-STAMP via the expression of RANKL.

In 2006, we reported that antibodies against CD47 expressed on monocytes inhibits human osteoclastogenesis by blocking monocyte fusion [72]. CD47, widely expressed on hematopoietic cells, is a ligand for monocyte/macrophage adhesion and fusion leading to multinucleation. We demonstrated as follows: 1) CD47 is expressed on monocytes but not on osteoclasts; 2) adding anti-CD47 antibody during day 0-3 of the culture period markedly inhibited osteoclastogenesis compared with adding anti-CD47 antibody during days 4-6; and 3)there was a tendency that in total CD14+ monocytes from PBMC, the mean of fluorescence intensity (MFI) on CD47+ cell was higher in patients with RA than in healthy controls [72]. Recently, another group also reported that osteoclast formation is strongly reduced both in vivo and in vitro in the absence of CD47/signal regulatory protein alpha (SIRPα) interaction using blocking antibodies *in vitro* and CD47-/- mice *in vivo* [73]. Thus, these and our findings suggest that CD47 could be a therapeutic target for bone destruction in RA.

7. Dexamethasone

Therapies using systemic glucocorticoid induce osteoporosis as a serious complication; however, the mechanism of glucocorticoid-induced osteoporosis remains unclear. It has been reported that glucocorticoids promote osteoclastogenesis by inhibiting OPG and concurrently stimulating RANKL production by osteoblastic lineage cells [74,75]. In addition, dexamethasone increases the pit area by human osteoclasts induced from monocytes stimulated by RANKL [75]. Thus, glucocorticoids induce osteoporosis both dependently on and independently of osteoblasts.

We hypothesized that activated human T cells are involved in glucocorticoid-induced osteoporosis. We have demonstrated that using human PBMC culture, dexamethasone stimulates osteoclastogenesis by elevating the RANKL-to-IFN-γ ratio expressed on human CD4+ T cells, which is inhibited by adding OPG [76]. Thus, it is suggested that human T cells stimulated by glucocorticoids, at least in part, play a role in human glucocorticoid-induced osteoporosis.

8. Tacrolimus

Tacrolimus (FK506) has been shown to have an optimally anti-inflammatory effect against patients with RA. Tacrolimus diminishes the ability of calcineurin to translocate the nuclear factor of activated T cells (NFAT) that initiates gene transcription for the synthesis of inflammatory cytokines [77]; however, the effect of tacrolimus on human osteoclastogenesis remains unclear.

We have demonstrated that tacrolimus dose-dependently inhibits dexamethasone-induced osteoclastogenesis from human PBMC [78]. As mentioned above, dexamethasone induces human osteoclastogenesis from PBMC, stimulating osteoclastogenesis by elevating the RANKL-to-IFN-γ ratio expressed on human CD4+ T cells [76]. The expression of RANKL stimulated by dexamethasone was markedly reduced by adding tacrolimus [78]. Thus, tacrolimus indirectly inhibited human osteoclastogenesis from PBMC induced by dexamethasone.

On the other hand, tacrolimus directly inhibits osteoclastogenesis. Igarashi et al. reported that FK506 directly induces osteoclast apoptosis in mouse bone marrow cultures [79]. In addition, Miyazaki et al. demonstrated that tacrolimus directly inhibits human osteoclastogenesis via targeting the calcineurin-dependent NFAT pathway and an activation pathway for c-Jun or microphthalmia transcription factor (MITF) in rheumatoid arthritis [80]. Moreover, it has been reported that tacrolimus administration into mice blocks osteclast differentiation, although the administration induces the reduction of bone mass, causing severe impairment of bone formation [81]. Thus, tacrolimus inhibits osteoclastogenesis both directly and indirectly.

9. Single Nucleotide Polymorphism (SNP)

The association of SNPs in RANKL with bone mineral density has been reported [82-84]. In addition, Wu et al. have reported that novel RANKL polymorphisms are associated with an earlier age at RA onset in shared epitope (SE)+, but not SE-, patients and that an interaction between SE-containing HLA-DRB1 and RANKL polymorphisms increases disease penetrance, resulting in a mean age at RA onset that is 18-20 years younger [85]. On the other hand, the association of SNPs in IL-17F with asthma and no significant association in IL-17A and F in osteoarthritis has been reported [86,87], whereas the association of SNPs in IL-17A or F with bone mineral density or RA has not been reported. In addition, a highly significant association between Crohn's disease and the IL-23 receptor gene was found; an uncommon coding variant confers strong protection against Crohn's disease [88]. Replication studies confirmed IL-23 receptor associations in independent cohorts of patients with Crohn's disease or ulcerative colitis [88]. However, the association of SNPs in IL-23 or IL-23 receptor with RA has not been reported.

In 2004, we have demonstrated that SNPs in RANKL and IL-17A genes are significantly associated with radiographic progression after 2 years in patients with early RA [89]. Thus, bone resorption induced by activated T cells may be genetically regulated through SNPs in RANKL and IL-17 in T cells; however, further investigation is necessary to clarify the association using a large number of patients for longer duration.

Conclusion

The role of T cells on human osteoclastogenesis has been clarified in vitro. However, the function of Th1 cells and Th17 cells on bone resorption has not fully been understood in humans including patients with RA, while Th1 cells and Th17 cells have been demonstrated to stimulate bone resorption in a murine model *in vivo*. Thus, further investigation is necessary to clarify the role of Th1 cells and Th17 cells in bone resorption of human diseases including RA.

Acknowledgments

We thank Dr. Nobuo Nara (Tokyo Medical and Dental University) for providing helpful suggestions regarding human hematopoiesis, and Ms. Hanae Kikuchi (Tokyo Women's Medical University) for her excellent experimental technique.

References

[1] Motoyoshi, K., Suda, T., Kusumoto, K., Takaku, F. & Miura, Y. (1982). Granulocyte-macrophage colony-stimulating and binding activities of purified human urinary

colony-stimulating factor to murine and human bone marrow cells. *Blood*, *60*, 1378-1386.

[2] Kanamaru, F., Iwai, H., Ikeda, T., Nakajima, A., Ishikawa, I. & Azuma, M. (2004). Expression of membrane-bound and soluble receptor activator of NF-kappaB ligand (RANKL) in human T cells. *Immunol Lett*, *94*, 239-246.

[3] Baecher-Allan, C., Brown, J. A., Freeman, G. J. & Hafler, D. A. (2001). CD4+CD25high regulatory cells in human peripheral blood. *J Immunol*, *167*, 1245-1253.

[4] Valencia, X., Stephens, G., Goldbach-Mansky, R., Wilson, M., Shevach, E. M. & Lipsky, P. E. (2006). TNF downmodulates the function of human CD4+CD25hi T-regulatory cells. *Blood*, *108*, 253-261.

[5] Amadi-Obi, A., Yu, C.R., Liu, X., Mahdi, R. M., Clarke, G. L., Nussenblatt, R. B., Gery, I., Lee, Y. S. & Egwuagu, C. E. (2007). T(H)17 cells contribute to uveitis and scleritis and are expanded by IL-2 and inhibited by IL-27/STAT1. *Nat Med*, May 13; [Epub ahead of print]

[6] Kotake, S., Nanke, Y., Mogi, M., Kawamoto, M., Furuya, T., Yago, T., Kobashigawa, T., Togari, A. & Kamatani. (2005). IFN-gamma-producing human T cells directly induce osteoclastogenesis from human monocytes via the expression of RANKL. *Eur J Immunol*, *35*, 3353-3363.

[7] Geusens, P. P., Landewe, R. B., Garnero, P., Chen, D., Dunstan, C. R., Lems, W. F., Stinissen, P., van der Heijde, D. M., van der Linden, S. & Boers, M. (2006). The ratio of circulating osteoprotegerin to RANKL in early rheumatoid arthritis predicts later joint destruction. *Arthritis Rheum*, *54*, 1772-1777.

[8] Luxenburg, C., Geblinger, D., Klein, E., Anderson, K., Hanein, D., Geiger, B. & Addadi L. (2007). The architecture of the adhesive apparatus of cultured osteoclasts: from podosome formation to sealing zone assembly. *PLoS ONE*, *2*, e179.

[9] Fuller, K., Kirstein, B. & Chambers, T. J. (2007). Regulation and enzymatic basis of bone resorption by human osteoclasts. *Clin Sci (Lond)*, *112*, 567-575.

[10] Shimizu, S., Shiozawa, S., Shiozawa, K., Imura, S. & Fujita, T. (1985). Quantitative histologic studies on the pathogenesis of periarticular osteoporosis in rheumatoid arthritis. *Arthritis Rheum*, *28*, 25-31.

[11] Kotake, S., Sato, K., Kim, K. J., Takahashi, N., Udagawa, N., Nakamura, I., Yamaguchi, A., Kishimoto, T., Suda, T. & Kashiwazaki, S. (1996). Interleukin-6 and soluble interleukin-6 receptors in the synovial fluids from rheumatoid arthritis patients are responsible for osteoclast-like cell formation. *J Bone Miner Res.*, *11*, 88-95.

[12] Kotake, S., Higaki, M., Sato, K., Himeno, S., Morita, H., Kim, K. J., Nara, N., Miyasaka, N., Nishioka, K. & Kashiwazaki, S. (1992). Detection of myeloid precursors (granulocyte/macrophage colony forming units) in the bone marrow adjacent to rheumatoid arthritis joints. *J Rheumatol*, *19*, 1511-1516.

[13] Kotake, S., Schumacher, H. R., Jr, Yarboro, C. H., Arayssi, T. K., Pando, J. A., Kanik, K. S., Gourley, M. F., Klippel, J. H. & Wilder, R. L. (1997). In vivo gene expression of type 1 and type 2 cytokines in synovial tissues from patients in early stages of rheumatoid, reactive, and undifferentiated arthritis. *Proc Assoc Am Physicians.*, *109*, 286-301. *Proc Assoc Am Physicians*, *109*, 286-301.

[14] Kotake, S., Schumacher, H. R., Jr, Arayssi, T. K., Gerard, H. C., Branigan, P. J., Hudson A. P., Yarboro, C. H., Klippel, J. H. & Wilder, R. L. (1999). Gamma interferon

and interleukin-10 gene expression in synovial tissues from patients with early stages of Chlamydia-associated arthritis and undifferentiated oligoarthritis and from healthy volunteers. *Infect Immun*, *67*, 2682-2686.

[15] Kotake, S., Schumacher, H. R. Jr, & Wilder, R. L. (1996). A simple nested RT-PCR method for quantitation of the relative amounts of multiple cytokine mRNAs in small tissue samples. *J Immunol Methods*, *199*, 193-203.

[16] Takahashi, N., Akatsu, T., Udagawa, N., Sasaki, T., Yamaguchi, A., Moseley, J. M., Martin, T. J. & Suda, T. (1988). Osteoblastic cells are involved in osteoclast formation. *Endocrinology*, *123*, 2600-2602.

[17] Udagawa, N., Takahashi, N., Akatsu, T., Tanaka, H., Sasaki, T., Nishihara, T., Koga, T., Martin, T. J. & Suda, T. (1990). Origin of osteoclasts: mature monocytes and macrophages are capable of differentiating into osteoclasts under a suitable microenvironment prepared by bone marrow-derived stromal cells. *Proc Natl Acad Sci U S A*, *87*, 7260-7264.

[18] Suda, T., Udagawa, N., Nakamura, I., Miyaura, C. & Takahashi, N. (1995). Modulation of osteoclast differentiation by local factors. *Bone*, *17*(2 Suppl), 87S-91S.

[19] Udagawa, N., Kotake, S., Kamatani, N., Takahashi, N. & Suda, T. (2002). The molecular mechanism of osteoclastogenesis in rheumatoid arthritis. *Arthritis Res.*, *4*, 281-289.

[20] Lam, J., Nelson, C. A., Ross, F. P., Teitelbaum, S. L. & Fremont, D. H. (2001). Crystal structure of the TRANCE/RANKL cytokine reveals determinants of receptor-ligand specificity. *J Clin Invest*, *108*, 971-979.

[21] Kong, Y. Y., Feige, U., Sarosi, I., Bolon, B., Tafuri, A., Morony, S., Capparelli, C., Li, J., Elliott, R., McCabe, S., Wong, T., Campagnuolo, G., Moran, E., Bogoch, E. R., Van, G., Nguyen, L. T., Ohashi, P. S., Lacey, D. L., Fish, E., Boyle, W. J. & Penninger, J. M. (1999). Activated T cells regulate bone loss and joint destruction in adjuvant arthritis through osteoprotegerin ligand. *Nature*, *402*, 304-309.

[22] Horwood, N. J., Kartsogiannis, V., Quinn, J. M., Romas, E., Martin, T. J. & Gillespie, M. T. (1999). Activated T lymphocytes support osteoclast formation in vitro. *Biochem Biophys Res Commun*, *265*, 144-150.

[23] Kotake, S., Udagawa, N., Hakoda, M., Mogi, M., Yano, K., Tsuda, E., Takahashi, K., Furuya, T., Ishiyama, S., Kim, K. J., Saito, S., Nishikawa, T., Takahashi, N., Togari, A., Tomatsu, T., Suda, T. & Kamatani, N. (2001). Activated human T cells directly induce osteoclastogenesis from human monocytes: possible role of T cells in bone destruction in rheumatoid arthritis patients. *Arthritis Rheum*, *44*, 1003-1012.

[24] Miranda-Carus, M. E., Benito-Miguel, M., Balsa, A., Cobo-Ibanez, T., Perez de Ayala, C., Pascual-Salcedo, D. & Martin-Mola, E. (2006). Peripheral blood T lymphocytes from patients with early rheumatoid arthritis express RANKL and interleukin-15 on the cell surface and promote osteoclastogenesis in autologous monocytes. *Arthritis Rheum.*, *54*, 1151-1164.

[25] Kobayashi, K., Takahashi, N., Jimi, E, Udagawa, N., Takami, M., Kotake, S., Nakagawa, N., Kinosaki, M., Yamaguchi, K., Shima, N., Yasuda, H., Morinaga, T., Higashio, K., Martin, T. J. & Suda, T. (2000). Tumor necrosis factor alpha stimulates osteoclast differentiation by a mechanism independent of the ODF/RANKL-RANK interaction. *J Exp Med*, *191*, 275-286.

[26] Mogi, M., Otogoto, J., Ota, N. & Togari, A. (2004). Differential expression of RANKL and osteoprotegerin in gingival crevicular fluid of patients with periodontitis. *J Dent Res.*, *83*, 166-169.
[27] Vernal, R., Dutzan, N., Hernandez, M., Chandia, S., Puente, J., Leon, R., Garcia, L., Del Valle, I., Silva, A. & Gamonal, J. (2006). High expression levels of receptor activator of nuclear factor-kappa B ligand associated with human chronic periodontitis are mainly secreted by CD4+ T lymphocytes. *J Periodontol*, *77*, 1772-1780.
[28] Teng, Y. T., Nguyen, H., Gao, X., Kong, Y. Y., Gorczynski, R. M., Singh, B., Ellen, R. P. & Penninger, J. M. (2000). Functional human T-cell immunity and osteoprotegerin ligand control alveolar bone destruction in periodontal infection. *J Clin Invest.*, *106*, R59-67.
[29] Kawai, T., Paster, B. J., Komatsuzawa, H., Ernst, C. W., Goncalves, R. B., Sasaki, H., Ouhara, K., Stashenko, P. P., Sugai, M. & Taubman, M. A. (2007). Cross-reactive adaptive immune response to oral commensal bacteria results in an induction of receptor activator of nuclear factor-kappaB ligand (RANKL)-dependent periodontal bone resorption in a mouse model. *Oral Microbiol Immunol*, *22*, 208-215.
[30] Rouvier, E., Luciani, M. F., Mattei, M. G., Denizot, F. & Golstein, P. (1993). CTLA-8, cloned from an activated T cell, bearing AU-rich messenger RNA instability sequences, and homologous to a herpesvirus saimiri gene. *J Immunol*, *150*, 5445-5456.
[31] Fossiez, F., Djossou, O., Chomarat, P., Flores-Romo, L., Ait-Yahia, S., Maat, C., Pin, J. J., Garrone, P., Garcia, E., Saeland, S., Blanchard, D., Gaillard, C., Das Mahapatra, B., Rouvier, E., Golstein, P., Banchereau, J. & Lebecque, S. (1996). T cell interleukin-17 induces stromal cells to produce proinflammatory and hematopoietic cytokines. *J Exp Med*, *183*, 2593-2603.
[32] Kotake, S. & Kamatani, N. (2002). The Role of IL-17 in Joint Destruction. *Drug News Perspect*, *15*, 17-23.
[33] Novatchkova, M., Leibbrandt, A., Werzowa, J., Neubuser, A. & Eisenhaber, F. (2003). The STIR-domain superfamily in signal transduction, development and immunity. *Trends Biochem Sci.*, *28*, 226-229.
[34] Maitra, A., Shen, F., Hanel, W., Mossman, K., Tocker, J., Swart, D. & Gaffen, S. L. (2007). Distinct functional motifs within the IL-17 receptor regulate signal transduction and target gene expression. *Proc Natl Acad Sci U S A*, *104*, 7506-7511.
[35] Kolls, J. K. & Linden, A. (2004). Interleukin-17 family members and inflammation. *Immunity*, *21*, 467-476.
[36] Toy, D., Kugler, D., Wolfson, M., van den Bos, T., Gurgel, J., Derry, J., Tocker, J. & Peschon, J. (2006). Interleukin 17 signals through a heteromeric receptor complex. *J Immunol*, *177*, 36-39.
[37] Kotake, S., Udagawa, N., Takahashi, N., Matsuzaki, K., Itoh, K., Ishiyama, S., Saito, S., Inoue, K., Kamatani, N., Gillespie, M. T., Martin, T. J. & Suda, T. (1999). IL-17 in synovial fluids from patients with rheumatoid arthritis is a potent stimulator of osteoclastogenesis. *J Clin Invest*, *103*, 1345-1352.
[38] Yago, T., Nanke, Y., Furuya, T., Kobashigawa, T., Kamatani, N. & Kotake, S. (2004). Infliximab potently inhibits osteoclastogenesis from human monocytes alone induced by IL-17 in the absence of osteoblasts. *Arthritis Rheum 50 (supple)*, *662*, S289 (abst).

[39] Lam, J., Takeshita, S., Barker, J. E., Kanagawa, O., Ross, F. P. & Teitelbaum, S. L. (2000). TNF-alpha induces osteoclastogenesis by direct stimulation of macrophages exposed to permissive levels of RANK ligand. *J Clin Invest.*, *106*, 1481-1488.

[40] Zou, W., Hakim, I., Tschoep, K., Endres, S. & Bar-Shavit, Z. (2001). Tumor necrosis factor-alpha mediates RANK ligand stimulation of osteoclast differentiation by an autocrine mechanism. *J Cell Biochem*, *83*, 70-83.

[41] Lubberts, E., Koenders, M. I., Oppers-Walgreen, B., van den Bersselaar, L., Coenen-de Roo, C. J., Joosten, L. A. & van den Berg, W. B. (2004). Treatment with a neutralizing anti-murine interleukin-17 antibody after the onset of collagen-induced arthritis reduces joint inflammation, cartilage destruction, and bone erosion. *Arthritis Rheum*, *50*, 650-659.

[42] Kotake, S. (2002). The role of IL-17 in joint destruction. *The 11th International Rheumatology Symposium in Kobe*, IS2-1 (abst).

[43] Nakae, S., Saijo, S., Horai, R., Sudo, K., Mori, S. & Iwakura, Y. (2003). IL-17 production from activated T cells is required for the spontaneous development of destructive arthritis in mice deficient in IL-1 receptor antagonist. *Proc Natl Acad Sci USA*, *100*, 5986-5990.

[44] Sarkar, S., Tesmer, L. A., Hindnavis, V., Endres, J. L. & Fox, D. A. (2007). Interleukin-17 as a molecular target in immune-mediated arthritis: immunoregulatory properties of genetically modified murine dendritic cells that secrete interleukin-4. *Arthritis Rheum*, *56*, 89-100.

[45] Raza, K., Falciani, F., Curnow, S. J., Ross, E. J., Lee, C. Y., Akbar, A. N., Lord, J. M., Gordon, C., Buckley, C. D. & Salmon, M. (2005). Early rheumatoid arthritis is characterized by a distinct and transient synovial fluid cytokine profile of T cell and stromal cell origin. *Arthritis Res Ther.*, *7*, R784-795.

[46] Murphy, C. A., Langrish, C. L., Chen, Y., Blumenschein, W., McClanahan, T., Kastelein, R. A., Sedgwick, J. D. & Cua, D. J. (2003). Divergent pro- and antiinflammatory roles for IL-23 and IL-12 in joint autoimmune inflammation. *J Exp Med*, *198*, 1951-1957.

[47] Yago, T., Nanke, Y., Kawamoto, M., Furuya, T., Kobashigawa, T., Kamatani, N. & Kotake, S. (2005). Interleukin-23 induces human osteoclastogenesis in vitro, and anti-interleukin-23 antibody reduces joint inflammation in rats with collagen-induced arthritis. *Arthritis Rheum. 52* (supple), 1309, S496 (abst).

[48] Mosmann, T. R., Cherwinski, H., Bond, M. W., Giedlin, M. A. & Coffman, R. L. (1986). Two types of murine helper T cell clone. I. Definition according to profiles of lymphokine activities and secreted proteins. *J Immunol*, *136*, 2348-2357.

[49] Furuzawa-Carballeda, J., Vargas-Rojas, M. I. & Cabral, A. R. (2007). Autoimmune inflammation from the Th17 perspective. *Autoimmun Rev.*, *6*, 169-175.

[50] Harrington, L. E., Hatton, R. D., Mangan, P. R., Turner, H., Murphy, T. L., Murphy, K. M. & Weaver, C. T. (2005). Interleukin 17-producing CD4+ effector T cells develop via a lineage distinct from the T helper type 1 and 2 lineages. *Nat Immunol*, *6*, 1123-1132.

[51] Park, H., Li, Z., Yang, X. O., Chang, S. H., Nurieva, R., Wang, Y. H., Wang, Y., Hood, L., Zhu, Z., Tian, Q. & Dong, C. (2005). A distinct lineage of CD4 T cells regulates tissue inflammation by producing interleukin 17. *Nat Immunol*, *6*, 1133-1141.

[52] Veldhoen, M., Hocking, R. J., Atkins, C. J., Locksley, R. M. & Stockinger, B. (2006). TGFbeta in the context of an inflammatory cytokine milieu supports de novo differentiation of IL-17-producing T cells. *Immunity*, *24*, 179-89.

[53] Bettelli, E., Carrier, Y., Gao, W., Korn, T., Strom, T. B., Oukka, M., Weiner, H. L. & Kuchroo, V. K. (2006). Reciprocal developmental pathways for the generation of pathogenic effector TH17 and regulatory T cells. *Nature*, *441*, 235-238.

[54] Mangan, P. R., Harrington, L. E., O'Quinn, D. B., Helms, W. S., Bullard, D. C., Elson, C. O., Hatton, R. D., Wahl, S. M., Schoeb, T. R. & Weaver, C. T. (2006). Transforming growth factor-beta induces development of the T(H)17 lineage. *Nature*, *441*, 231-234.

[55] Acosta-Rodriguez, E. V., Rivino, L., Geginat, J., Jarrossay, D., Gattorno, M., Lanzavecchia, A., Sallusto, F. & Napolitani, G. (2007). Surface phenotype and antigenic specificity of human interleukin 17-producing T helper memory cells. *Nat Immunol*, *8*, 639-646.

[56] Ye, P., Rodriguez, F. H., Kanaly, S., Stocking, K. L., Schurr, J., Schwarzenberger, P., Oliver, P., Huang, W., Zhang, P., Zhang, J., Shellito, J. E., Bagby, G. J., Nelson, S., Charrier, K., Peschon, J. J. & Kolls, J. K. (2001). Requirement of interleukin 17 receptor signaling for lung CXC chemokine and granulocyte colony-stimulating factor expression, neutrophil recruitment, and host defense. *J Exp Med*, *194*, 519-527.

[57] Happel, K. I., Dubin, P. J., Zheng, M., Ghilardi, N., Lockhart, C., Quinton, L. J., Odden, A. R., Shellito, J. E., Bagby, G. J., Nelson, S. & Kolls, J. K. (2005). Divergent roles of IL-23 and IL-12 in host defense against Klebsiella pneumoniae. *J Exp Med*, *202*, 761-769.

[58] Rudner, X. L., Happel, K. I., Young, E. A. & Shellito, J. E. (2007). Interleukin-23 (IL-23)-IL-17 Cytokine Axis in Murine Pneumocystis carinii Infection. *Infect Immun*, *75*, 3055-3061.

[59] Sato, K., Suematsu, A., Okamoto, K., Yamaguchi, A., Morishita, Y., Kadono, Y., Tanaka, S., Kodama, T., Akira, S., Iwakura, Y., Cua, D. J. & Takayanagi, H. (2006). Th17 functions as an osteoclastogenic helper T cell subset that links T cell activation and bone destruction. *J Exp Med*, *203*, 2673-2682.

[60] Hirota, K., Hashimoto, M., Yoshitomi, H., Tanaka, S., Nomura, T., Yamaguchi, T., Iwakura, Y., Sakaguchi, N. & Sakaguchi, S. (2007). T cell self-reactivity forms a cytokine milieu for spontaneous development of IL-17+ Th cells that cause autoimmune arthritis. *J Exp Med*, *204*, 41-47.

[61] Takahashi, K., Azuma, T., Motohira, H., Kinane, D. F. & Kitetsu, S. (2005). The potential role of interleukin-17 in the immunopathology of periodontal disease. *J Clin Periodontol*, *32*, 369-374.

[62] Oda, T., Yoshie, H. & Yamazaki, K. (2003). Porphyromonas gingivalis antigen preferentially stimulates T cells to express IL-17 but not receptor activator of NF-kappaB ligand in vitro. *Oral Microbiol Immunol*, *18*, 30-36.

[63] Fox, S. W., Fuller, K., Bayley, K. E, Lean, J. M. & Chambers, T. J. (2000). TGF-beta 1 and IFN-gamma direct macrophage activation by TNF-alpha to osteoclastic or cytocidal phenotype. *J Immunol*, *165*, 4957-4963.

[64] Udagawa, N., Horwood, N. J., Elliott, J., Mackay, A., Owens, J., Okamura, H., Kurimoto, M., Chambers, T. J., Martin, T. J. & Gillespie, M. T. (1997). Interleukin-18 (interferon-gamma-inducing factor) is produced by osteoblasts and acts via

granulocyte/macrophage colony-stimulating factor and not via interferon-gamma to inhibit osteoclast formation. *J Exp Med., 185*, 1005-1012.

[65] Takayanagi, H., Ogasawara, K., Hida, S., Chiba, T., Murata, S., Sato, K., Takaoka, A., Yokochi, T., Oda, H., Tanaka, K., Nakamura, K. & Taniguchi, T. (2000). T-cell-mediated regulation of osteoclastogenesis by signalling cross-talk between RANKL and IFN-gamma. *Nature, 408*, 600-605.

[66] Gao, Y., Grassi, F., Ryan, M. R., Terauchi, M., Page, K., Yang, X., Weitzmann, M. N. & Pacifici, R. (2007). IFN-gamma stimulates osteoclast formation and bone loss in vivo via antigen-driven T cell activation. *J Clin Invest, 117*, 122-132.

[67] Stashenko, P., Goncalves, R. B., Lipkin, B., Ficarelli, A., Sasaki, H. & Campos-Neto, A. (2007). Th1 immune response promotes severe bone resorption caused by Porphyromonas gingivalis. *Am J Pathol, 170*, 203-213.

[68] Kim, Y. G., Lee, C. K., Nah, S. S., Mun, S. H., Yoo, B. & Moon, H. B. (2007). Human CD4+CD25+ regulatory T cells inhibit the differentiation of osteoclasts from peripheral blood mononuclear cells. *Biochem Biophys Res Commun*, 357, 1046-1052.

[69] Hartgers, F. C., Vissers, J. L., Looman, M. W., van Zoelen, C., Huffine, C., Figdor, C. G. & Adema, G. J. (2000). DC-STAMP, a novel multimembrane-spanning molecule preferentially expressed by dendritic cells. *Eur J Immunol, 30*, 3585-3590.

[70] Kukita, T., Wada, N., Kukita, A., Kakimoto, T., Sandra, F., Toh, K., Nagata, K., Iijima, T., Horiuchi, M., Matsusaki, H., Hieshima, K., Yoshie, O. & Nomiyama, H. (2004). RANKL-induced DC-STAMP is essential for osteoclastogenesis. *J Exp Med, 200*, 941-946.

[71] Yagi, M., Miyamoto, T., Sawatani, Y., Iwamoto, K., Hosogane, N., Fujita, N., Morita, K., Ninomiya, K., Suzuki, T., Miyamoto, K., Oike, Y., Takeya, M., Toyama, Y. & Suda, T. (2005). DC-STAMP is essential for cell-cell fusion in osteoclasts and foreign body giant cells. *J Exp Med, 202*, 345-351.

[72] Yago, T., Nanke, Y., Kawamoto, M., Furuya, T., Kobashigawa, T., Ichikawa, N., Kamatani, N. & Kotake, S. (2006). Antibodies against CD47 expressed on monocytes in rheumatoid arthritis patients inhibits human osteoclastogenesis by blocking fusion of monocytes. *Arthritis Rheum, 50* (supple), 1394, S354 (abst).

[73] Lundberg, P., Koskinen, C., Baldock, P. A., Lothgren, H., Stenberg, A., Lerner, U. H. & Oldenborg, P. A. (2007). Osteoclast formation is strongly reduced both in vivo and in vitro in the absence of CD47/SIRPalpha-interaction. *Biochem Biophys Res Commun, 352*, 444-448.

[74] Hofbauer, L. C., Gori, F., Riggs, B. L., Lacey, D. L., Dunstan, C. R., Spelsberg, T. C. & Khosla, S. (1999). Stimulation of osteoprotegerin ligand and inhibition of osteoprotegerin production by glucocorticoids in human osteoblastic lineage cells: potential paracrine mechanisms of glucocorticoid-induced osteoporosis. *Endocrinology, 140*, 4382-4389.

[75] Sivagurunathan, S., Muir, M. M., Brennan, T. C., Seale, J. P. & Mason, R. S. (2005). Influence of glucocorticoids on human osteoclast generation and activity. *J Bone Miner Res., 20*, 390-398.

[76] Yago, T., Nanke, Y., Kawamoto, M., Furuya, T., Kobashigawa, T., Kamatani, N. & Kotake, S. (2006). Dexamethasone directly induce osteoclastogenesis from human PBMC by elevating the RANKL-to-IFN-γ ratio on T cells even in the absence of

osteoblasts. –possible mechanism of corticosteroids in inducing osteoporosis-. *Arthritis Rheum. 50* (supple), *1277*, S531 (abst).

[77] Kitahara, K. & Kawai, S. (2007). Cyclosporine and tacrolimus for the treatment of rheumatoid arthritis. *Curr Opin Rheumatol*, *19*, 238-245.

[78] Yago, T., Nanke, Y., Kawamoto, M., Furuya, T., Kobashigawa, T., Kamatani, N. & Kotake, S. (2006). Tacrolimus potently inhibits dexamethasone-induced osteoclastogenesis from human PBMC. – possible role of tacrolimus in preventing bone destruction. *Arthritis Rheum. 50* (supple), 1393, S354 (abst).

[79] Igarashi, K., Hirotani, H., Woo, J. T. & Stern, P. H. (2004). Cyclosporine A and FK506 induce osteoclast apoptosis in mouse bone marrow cell cultures. *Bone*, *35*, 47-56.

[80] Miyazaki, M., Fujikawa, Y., Takita, C. & Tsumura, H. (2007). Tacrolimus and cyclosporine A inhibit human osteoclast formation via targeting the calcineurin-dependent NFAT pathway and an activation pathway for c-Jun or MITF in rheumatoid arthritis. *Clin Rheumatol*, *26*, 231-239.

[81] Koga, T., Matsui, Y., Asagiri, M., Kodama, T., de Crombrugghe, B., Nakashima, K. & Takayanagi, H. (2005). NFAT and Osterix cooperatively regulate bone formation. *Nat Med*, *11*, 880-885.

[82] Xiong, D. H., Shen, H., Zhao, L. J., Xiao, P., Yang, T. L., Guo, Y., Wang, W., Guo, Y. F., Liu, Y. J., Recker, R. R. & Deng, H. W. (2006). Robust and comprehensive analysis of 20 osteoporosis candidate genes by very high-density single-nucleotide polymorphism screen among 405 white nuclear families identified significant association and gene-gene interaction. *J Bone Miner Res.*, *21*, 1678-1695.

[83] Mencej, S., Prezelj, J., Kocijancic, A., Ostanek, B. & Marc, J. (2006). Association of TNFSF11 gene promoter polymorphisms with bone mineral density in postmenopausal women. *Maturitas*, *55*, 219-226.

[84] Hsu, Y. H., Niu, T., Terwedow, H. A., Xu, X., Feng, Y., Li, Z., Brain, J. D., Rosen, C. J., Laird, N. & Xu, X. (2006). Variation in genes involved in the RANKL/RANK/OPG bone remodeling pathway are associated with bone mineral density at different skeletal sites in men. *Hum Genet*, *118*, 568-577.

[85] Wu, H., Khanna, D., Park, G., Gersuk, V., Nepom, G. T., Wong, W. K., Paulus, H. E. & Tsao, B. P. (2004). Interaction between RANKL and HLA-DRB1 genotypes may contribute to younger age at onset of seropositive rheumatoid arthritis in an inception cohort. *Arthritis Rheum*, *50*, 3093-3103.

[86] Kawaguchi, M., Takahashi, D., Hizawa, N., Suzuki, S., Matsukura, S., Kokubu, F., Maeda, Y., Fukui, Y., Konno, S., Huang, S. K., Nishimura, M. & Adachi, M. R. (2006). IL-17F sequence variant (His161Arg) is associated with protection against asthma and antagonizes wild-type IL-17F activity. *J Allergy Clin Immunol*, *117*, 795-801.

[87] Southam, L., Heath, O., Chapman, K. & Loughlin, J. (2006). Association analysis of the interleukin 17 genes IL17A and IL17F as potential osteoarthritis susceptibility loci. *Ann Rheum Dis.*, *65*, 556-557.

[88] Duerr, R. H., Taylor, K. D., Brant, S. R., Rioux, J. D., Silverberg, M. S., Daly, M. J., Steinhart, A. H., Abraham, C., Regueiro, M., Griffiths, A., Dassopoulos, T., Bitton, A., Yang, H., Targan, S., Datta, L. W., Kistner, E. O., Schumm, L. P., Lee, A. T., Gregersen, P. K., Barmada, M. M., Rotter, J. I., Nicolae, D. L. & Cho, J. H. (2006). A genome-wide association study identifies IL23R as an inflammatory bowel disease gene. *Science*, *314*, 1461-1463.

[89] Furuya, T., Ichikawa, N., Kogame, A., Nanke, Y., Higami, K., Hakoda, M., Kamatani, N. & Kotake, S. (2004). Association of polymorphisms in the receptor activator of nuclear factor-kappa B (RANK), RANK ligand, osteoprotegerin, and interleukin 17 genes with disease severity in Japanese patients with rheumatoid arthritis. *Arthritis Rheum*, *50*, (supple), 853, S354 (abst).

In: Rheumatoid Arthritis: Prevalence, Risk...
Editor: Michael H. Madsen

ISBN: 978-1-61761-931-1

Chapter 8

Subclinical Atherosclerosis in Patients with Rheumatoid and Psoriatic Arthritis

Elisabetta Profumo[1], Brigitta Buttari[1], Maria Elena Tosti[2], Rossana Scrivo[3], Antonio Spadaro[3], Chiara Tesori[4], Manuela Di Franco[3] and Rachele Riganò[1]

[1]Department of Infectious, Parasitic and Immune-mediated Diseases
[2]National Centre of Epidemiology, Surveillance and Health Promotion, Istituto Superiore di Sanità, Rome
[3] Rheumatology Unit
[4] Department of Surgical Sciences, University Sapienza, Rome, Italy.

Abstract

Accelerated development of atherosclerosis has been observed in patients with rheumatic diseases such as rheumatoid arthritis (RA) and psoriatic arthritis (PsA). It may be related to the inflammatory overload accompanied to the combination of an excessive production of reactive oxygen species with an impaired antioxidant defence capacity, leading to oxidative stress that may facilitate the development and progression of atherosclerosis. Compared with the general population, patients with RA die prematurely, mainly because of cardiovascular diseases but the mechanism by which premature atherosclerosis develops in RA is unknown. Recent data have demonstrated the prevalence of atherosclerosis also in patients with PsA, a chronic inflammatory autoimmune disease characterized by inflammatory arthritis and skin psoriasis. PsA shares some phenotypic characteristics with RA, even though the synovial inflammation of PsA is characterized by less macrophage infiltration and increased vascularity in comparison to RA inflammation. The increased cardiovascular risk in PsA and RA suggests the need to treat the inflammatory process and to monitor traditional atherosclerotic risk factors in these pathologies.

The aim of our study was to evaluate whether increased oxidative stress may be associated to the presence of subclinical atherosclerosis in patients with RA and in patients with PsA. For this purpose we determined the levels of oxidized low density lipoproteins (ox-LDL) and of nitric oxide (NO) in the sera obtained from 19 patients with RA, 20 with PsA and 20 sex- and age-matched healthy controls. Patients with RA fulfilled the American College of Rheumatology criteria, and patients with PsA fulfilled the CASPAR criteria. In all patients we evaluated the activity and duration of the disease and classical risk factors for atherosclerosis. Our results showed higher levels of ox-LDL and lower levels of NO in sera from patients with RA and PsA than in sera from healthy controls. Notably, higher serum levels of ox-LDL were observed in patients with an intima-media thickness (IMT) >1 than in those with an IMT ≤ 1, and higher serum levels of NO in patients with an IMT ≤ 1 than in those with an IMT >1, in patients with RA and PsA. Our data suggest that monitoring circulating levels of ox-LDL and NO in patients with RA and PsA could give information on the development of atherosclerotic disease and therefore could be useful to the clinical management of patients.

Introduction

Rheumatoid arthritis (RA) and psoriatic arthritis (PsA) are chronic inflammatory diseases of the musculoskeletal system. In RA the inflammatory process affects the synovium and leads to joint damage and bone destruction [1]. This pathology is characterised by significant morbidity as a result of synovial inflammation and associated disability [2]; it is more frequent in women than in men with a ratio 3:1. The tissue damage is primarily caused by immune complexes and by cell-mediated immunity. In patients affected by RA the synovial joints are characterized by an inflammatory infiltrate, mainly composed by T lymphocytes and monocytes that secrete soluble factors and promote Th1 inflammation, responsible for the tissue damage. Many studies have reported an excess of cardiovascular morbidity and mortality among patients with RA [2]. Compared with the general population, patients with RA die prematurely, mainly because of cardiovascular diseases. In patients with active disease, the majority of cardiovascular deaths are caused by accelerated atherosclerosis [3-6]. Atherosclerosis is a chronic inflammatory disease caused by endothelial dysfunction and characterized by complex interactions between immune and vascular cells. The activation of endothelial cells induces the expression of adhesion molecules on these cells and the recruitment of leucocytes, thus promoting the inflammatory response. Accelerated atherosclerosis observed in patients with RA is probably due to the chronic activation of inflammatory mechanisms involved in this pathology.

Psoriatic arthritis (PsA) is an inflammatory joint disease with heterogeneous presentation and clinical course [7]. Clear evidence exists that this disease is distinct from rheumatoid arthritis and other spondyloarthropathies, based on informations derived from characteristic clinical features, and on data from histopathologic analyses, immunogenetic associations and musculoskeletal imaging. It is usually seronegative for rheumatoid factor. PsA shares some phenotypic characteristics with RA, even though the synovial inflammation of PsA is characterized by less macrophage infiltration and increased vascularity in comparison to RA inflammation. Much interest has been focused previously on the prominent role of T lymphocytes in the inflammatory process; however, many studies strongly support a major contribution of macrophages in the initiation and perpetuation of joint and skin inflammation [7]. Recent data have demonstrated the occurrence of endothelial dysfunction and the prevalence of atherosclerosis also in patients with PsA [8,9]. The occurrence of cardiovascular disease might be directly linked to the cutaneous and musculoskeletal manifestations of this disease involving subsets of circulating monocytes and tissue macrophages activated by inflammatory mediators in the skin and joint [7].

As patients with autoimmune rheumatic diseases live longer due to improved therapies and preventive measures, mortality and disability due to cardiovascular diseases are increasing [10]. The relative risk to develop atherosclerosis is approximately 1.6 in PsA and 3.0 in RA. Increased risks are found when analyzed by atherosclerotic events, causes of death, or surrogate measures of atherosclerosis, such as carotid artery plaque, intima-media thickness (IMT), or coronary artery calcification. As RA and probably PsA predispose to atherosclerosis, an important issue is how to prevent this outcome. Therefore, when considering preventive interventions, the most important question is whether patients with some particular clinical features have greater risk for atherosclerosis. This may suggest that detecting a particular clinical marker will identify patients at high risk for clinical atherosclerosis and may help in establishing a risk prediction model. In the last decade great attention has been focused on the identification of risk factors predisposing to atherosclerotic diseases [11,12]. Many studies have demonstrated correlations of atherosclerosis with clinical conditions characterized by alteration in the metabolism such as diabetes [13] and hypercholesterolemia [14]. Gender is also a risk factor for cardiovascular diseases, as men have higher risk to develop atherosclerosis than women [15], and increasing age is associated with either clinical atherosclerotic events or surrogate markers for atherosclerosis, such as the occurrence of carotid plaque. Of particular interest are the well known associations of the standard measures of acute systemic inflammation such as erythrocyte sedimentation rate (ESR) [16], with atherosclerosis. Evidence exists suggesting that C-reactive protein (CRP) is a particularly consistent predictor of increased risk for atherosclerotic disease in the general population [17]. Traditional risk factors for atherosclerosis are operational in patients with autoimmune rheumatic diseases. Increased incidence of factors such as metabolic syndrome, diabetes and hypertension has been demonstrated in these patients. Furthermore, there may be genetic and environmental risk factors that predispose an individual both to autoimmune disease and to atherosclerosis. It is probably useful to consider certain autoimmune diseases, such as RA, to be equivalent to diabetes in increasing risk for developing atherosclerosis. Of note, among patients with autoimmune diseases, the interpretation of classical risk factors as CRP can be confounded by the correlation with the systemic inflammation that occurs in these pathologies. However, several studies have identified ESR as an independent risk factor for atherosclerosis in patients with RA.

Recently, accumulating evidence has demonstrated the presence of oxidative stress in patients with rheumatic diseases and suggested a role for the use of antioxidants in prevention and treatment of these pathologies [18,19]. It is well known that the inflammatory overload accompanied to the combination of an excessive production of reactive oxygen species with an impaired antioxidant defence capacity, leading to oxidative stress may facilitate the development and progression of atherosclerosis. Furthermore pharmacological control of oxidative stress and stimulation of nitric oxide release have proved to exert beneficial effects also on vascular remodeling in experimental diabetic models [20]. In several vascular disorders, an increase in superoxide (O_2^-) has been shown to contribute to reduced NO bioavailability through its reaction with NO to form peroxynitrite [21].

Thus, it is clear that the cellular redox state is dysregulated, and the resultant generation of reactive oxygen species (ROS) may play important role in driving and possibly initiating the rheumatic disease as well as cardiovascular complications. However, the precise mechanisms of ROS metabolism, and their function in the progression of these pathologies remain largely elusive.

The increased cardiovascular risk in PsA and RA suggests the need to treat the inflammatory process and to monitor traditional atherosclerotic risk factors in these pathologies.

Seeking more information on biomarkers for atherosclerosis development in patients with RA and PsA, in our in vitro study we evaluated the possible association of oxidative stress markers in peripheral blood with the presence of subclinical atherosclerosis. For this purpose, we determined by immune enzymatic assays serum levels of oxidized low density lipoproteins (ox-LDL) and NO in patients with RA and PsA divided into two groups according to the presence of atherosclerotic disease determined by echo-color Doppler ultrasonography. As controls we used healthy subjects free of atherosclerotic disease. We also investigated whether these two serum biomarkers were correlated to traditional risk factors for atherosclerosis or to clinical features of the two autoimmune diseases.

Materials and Methods

Study Population

We enrolled 19 consecutive patients with RA fulfilling the American College of Rheumatology (ACR) criteria [22] and 20 consecutive patients with PsA fulfilling the Classification Criteria for Psoriatic Arthritis (CASPAR) [23]. We also enrolled 20 sex- and age-matched healthy subjects as controls. Exclusion criteria for patients and controls were recent infection (< 1 month), other autoimmune diseases, malignancy and inflammatory diseases. In all patients we evaluated the activity and duration of the disease and classical risk factors for atherosclerosis (Table). None of the patients and healthy subjects had a history of cardiovascular manifestations. All patients were treated with disease-modifying antirheumatic drugs. Serum samples were obtained from patients and controls and stored at -80°C until use. Informed consent was obtained from all participants.

IMT of the Common Carotid Arteries

To evaluate the presence of atherosclerosis in patients and healthy subjects, IMT of the common carotid arteries was evaluated by Echo-color Doppler. Images were acquired on an ultrasound system equipped with a 7.5 MHz frequency linear-array transducer. The radiologist of the current study was blinded to RA and PsA patients and to the control group, and measurement of the IMT was always performed at the same arterial wall 1 cm proximal to the carotid bifurcation. Two parallel echogenic lines corresponding to the lumen/intima and media/adventitia interfaces were obtained. The distance between these 2 parallel lines corresponded to the IMT. Values were expressed in millimeters.

Table. Baseline Characteristics Of The 19 Patients With Rheumatoid Arthritis (RA) And Of The 20 Patients With Psoriatic Arthritis (Psa)

	Patients with RA	Patients with PsA	P[c]
N	19	20	
Age (years), median (range)	54 (30-64)	51 (35-69)	0.896
Male/female (n)	1/18	13/7	*<0.001*
Duration of the disease (years), median (range)	3 (0.5-25)	7 (1-24)	0.241
Smoking[a], n (%)	7 (37)	5 (25)	0.414
Hypertension[b], n (%)	4 (21)	2 (10)	0.374
Total cholesterol (mg/dl), median (range)	212.5 (160-257)	221 (153-296)	0.409
HDL cholesterol (mg/dl), median (range)	56.5 (45-74)	52 (30-76)	*0.028*
Triglycerids (mg/dl), median (range)	104.5 (90-166)	125 (93-566)	*0.018*
ESR, median (range)	18 (6-40)	10 (3-41)	*0.016*
CRP, median (range)	1.95 (0-43)	0 (0-16)	0.165
IMT >1, n (%)	9 (47)	11 (55)	0.271

a Smoking is defined as current smokers;

b Hypertension is defined as systolic blood pressure ≥140 mmHg, diastolic blood pressure ≥ 90 mm Hg, or need for hypertensive medication;

c Pearson's chi-squared test or Fisher exact test for discrete variables and Mann-Whitney test for continuous variables to evaluate the presence of a statistical significance among patients with RA and PsA;

ESR: erythrocyte sedimentation rate; CRP: C reactive protein; IMT: intima-media thickness.

Serum Ox-LDL and NO Levels

Ox-LDL and NO concentrations in serum samples from patients and healthy subjects were quantified with commercially available ELISA kits (Oxidized LDL Competitive ELISA, Mercodia, Uppsala, Sweden for ox-LDL; Nitrate/Nitrite Colorimetric Assay Kit, Cayman, Lausen Switzerland for NO), as recommended by the manufacturer. The detection limit of the assays were ≤ 0.3 U/L for ox-LDL, < 2.5 μM for NO.

Statistical Analysis

Data on serum ox-LDL and NO levels are expressed as medians and inter-quartile ranges. Mann-Whitney non parametric test was used to investigate the significance of unpaired continuous data. Pearson's chi-squared test or Fisher's exact test, when necessary, was used to evaluate the differences in discrete baseline characteristics between groups of patients. Correlations were explored by Spearman rank correlation coefficient. P values less than 0.05 were considered statistically significant.

All the statistical procedures were performed by STATA 8.1 statistical package.

Results

Serum Ox-LDL Levels in RA and PsA Patients

Patients with RA and PsA showed higher ox-LDL concentrations in serum compared to healthy subjects (Figure 1). No differences were observed between patients with RA and PsA in the ox-LDL mean level. When patients with RA and PsA were divided according to the IMT value obtained by Echo-color Doppler images, patients with IMT >1 showed higher levels of ox-LDL compared to patients with IMT ≤1 and to healthy subjects (Figure 2).

Serum NO Levels in RA and PsA Patients

Patients with RA and PsA showed lower NO levels in serum compared to healthy subjects (Figure 3). The difference resulted statistically significant for PsA (PsA, $P = 0.0155$; RA, $P = 0.0655$). In patients with RA and particularly with PsA, divided according to the IMT value by Echo-color Doppler images, NO levels were lower in patients with IMT >1 compared to patients with IMT ≤1 and to healthy subjects (Figure 4).

Association of Serum Ox-LDL and NO Levels with Baseline Characteristics of Patients

It is well known that there is a correlation among baseline clinical characteristics of patients and that these characteristics can be associated also to disease presentation. Analysis of association between risk factors and the autoimmune disease showed a significantly higher mean value of ESR and HDL-cholesterol in patients with AR than in patients with PsA ($P = 0.01$ and $P = 0.02$) (Table). In contrast the triglycerides value was significantly higher in patients with PsA than in patients with RA ($P = 0.0177$). In patients with RA, comparative analysis of risk factors with serum ox-LDL and NO levels showed a significant negative correlation between HDL-cholesterol and NO mean level ($r = -0.6$, $P = 0.013$) and a positive correlation near to the statistical significance between ox-LDL and cholesterol ($r = 0.5$, $P = 0.0528$). We did not find any correlation between traditional risk factors and the presence of subclinical atherosclerosis in patients with RA and PsA.

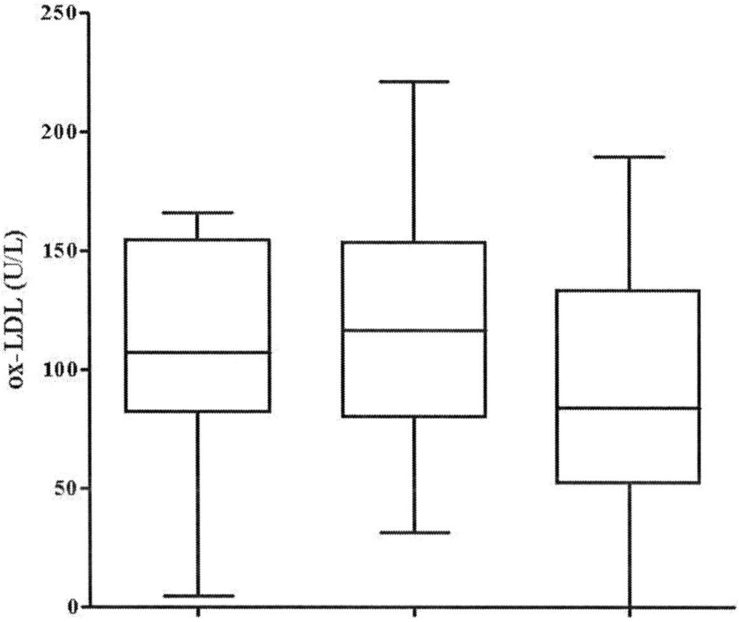

Figure 1. Box plot graphs showing oxidized LDL (ox-LDL) concentrations in serum samples from the 19 patients with rheumatoid arthritis (RA), the 20 patients with psoriatic arthritis (PsA) and the 20 healthy subjects. Patients with RA and PsA showed higher ox-LDL serum levels when compared to healthy subjects. No differences were observed between patients with RA and PsA

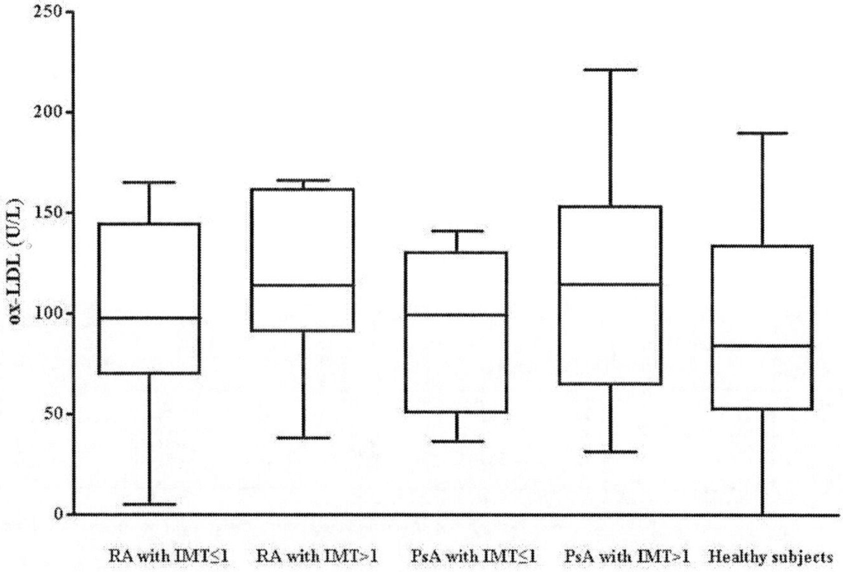

Figure 2. Box plot graphs showing oxidized LDL (ox-LDL) concentrations in serum samples from patients with rheumatoid arthritis (RA) and with psoriatic arthritis (PsA) divided according to the IMT value obtained by Echo-color Doppler images, and in serum samples from healthy subjects. Patients with RA and PsA showing an IMT >1 had higher levels of ox-LDL when compared to patients with IMT ≤1 and to healthy subjects.

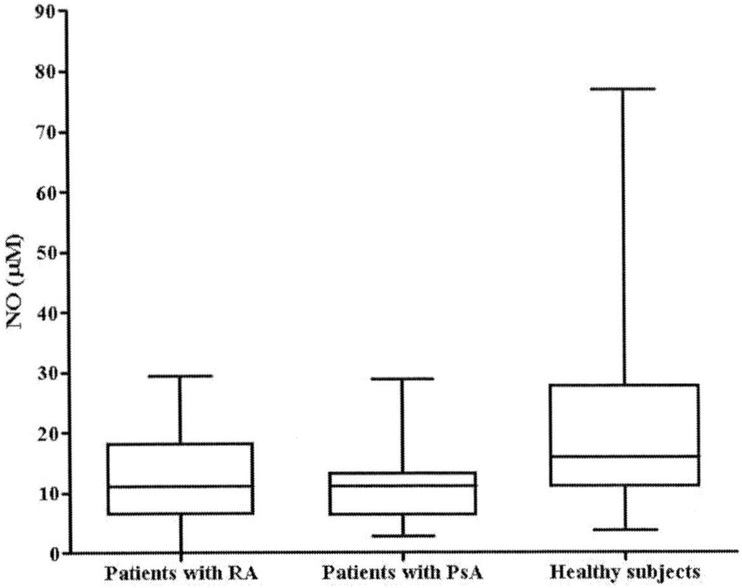

Figure 3. Box plot graphs showing nitric oxide (NO) concentrations in serum samples from the 19 patients with rheumatoid arthritis (RA), the 20 patients with psoriatic arthritis (PsA) and the 20 healthy subjects. Patients with RA and PsA showed lower NO serum levels when compared to healthy subjects. The difference resulted statistically significant for PsA (PsA, P =0.0155; RA, P = 0.0655)

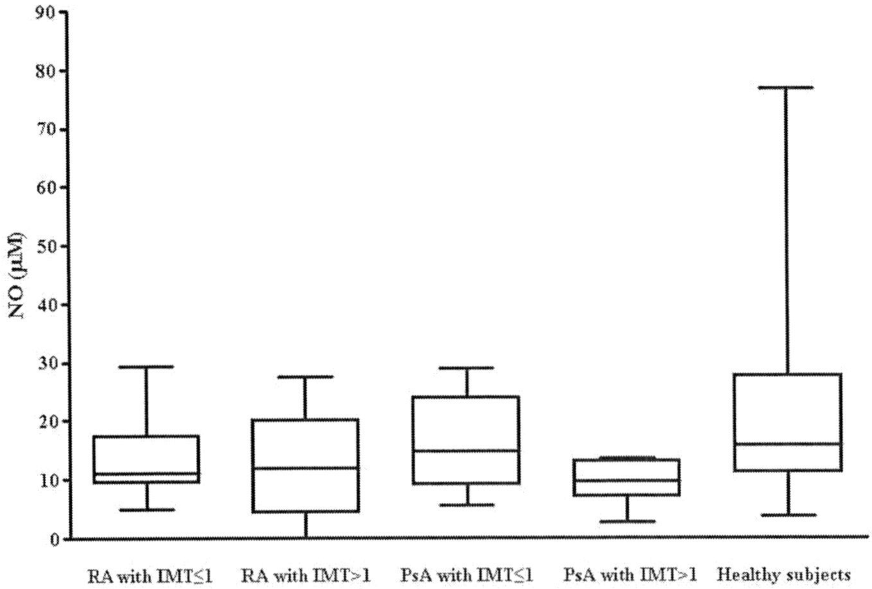

Figure 4. Box plot graphs showing nitric oxide (NO) concentrations in serum samples from patients with rheumatoid arthritis (RA) and with psoriatic arthritis (PsA) divided according to the IMT value obtained by Echo-color Doppler images, and in serum samples from healthy subjects. Patients with RA and PsA showing an IMT >1 had lower levels of NO when compared to patients with IMT ≤1 and to healthy subjects

Conclusion

Our preliminary findings reported in this chapter indicate that serum levels of ox-LDL and NO are putative biomarkers for atherosclerosis development in patients with RA and PsA. We found that serum ox-LDL levels, higher in patients with RA and PsA than in healthy subjects, were particularly higher in patients with subclinical atherosclerosis evaluated as IMT increase by Echo-color Doppler. In contrast serum NO levels resulted lower in patients with RA and PsA than in healthy subjects, particularly in patients with an increase in the IMT value (IMT >1). Our results of a negative association between ox-LDL and NO in patients are in line with previous findings indicating that ox-LDL impairs NO signaling and endothelial function thus contributing to the pathogenesis of atherosclerosis [24]. The endothelium plays a central role in overall vascular homeostasis by regulating vasoreactivity, platelet activation, leukocyte adhesion, and smooth muscle cell proliferation and migration. Endothelial NO, an important vasoprotective molecule, is a major modulator of these effects, and impaired NO signaling with associated endothelial activation is considered an early marker of the atherogenic process. Nitric oxide is produced by the action of endothelial NO synthase (eNOS), which uses L-arginine as its substrate [25]. However, L-arginine is also a substrate for arginase, which converts L-arginine to L-ornithine and urea [26]. Thus, substrate availability to, and thereby enzymatic products of either enzyme may be influenced by the activity and substrate utilization of the other. In human aortic endothelial cells, ox-LDL stimulation increases arginase enzyme activity in a time- and dose-dependent manner [27]. Thus, ox-LDLs increase arginase activity by a sequence of regulatory events, and this increased arginase activity contributes to ox-LDL-dependent impairment of NO production.

A limitation of our study is the low number of patients that probably does not allow to reach the statistical significance between the observed differences. The low number of patients also limits the possibility to find correlation of the two biomarkers evaluated in this study with traditional risk factors for atherosclerosis or clinical features of the rheumatic disease. Of note, in our study population the only statistically significant association was the negative correlation between NO and HDL-cholesterol levels in RA. Low levels of HDL cholesterol are usually recognized as an important independent risk factor for occurrence of cardiovascular events [28]. However, Agerholm-Larsen et al. observed an association of decreased HDL cholesterol levels with a paradoxical lower risk of ischemic heart disease in women [29]. These data suggest the hypothesis that the strong inverse association between HDL cholesterol concentrations and the occurrence of cardiovascular events observed in prospective epidemiological population studies is not due to HDL cholesterol levels per se, and that individuals with low HDL cholesterol may have a reduced risk of cardiovascular event occurrence. In the light of these previous data, it is not surprising the association between decreased levels of the vasoprotective mediator NO and increased concentrations of HDL cholesterol that we observed in patients with RA.

In conclusion, our study, although very preliminary and although not establishing a causal link between ox-LDL or NO levels and accelerated atherosclerosis, suggests that ox-LDL and NO levels may be operational as markers of atherosclerotic disease in patients with RA and PsA. The detection of circulating ox-LDL and NO levels in these patients might be a useful adjunct to imaging procedures as prognostic markers for the development of atherosclerotic disease and could be useful to the clinical management of patients. Clearly these interesting possibilities await confirmation in a larger number of patients.

References

[1] Haugeberg, G; Ørstavik, RE; Kvien, TK. Effects of rheumatoid arthritis on bone. Curr. Opin. *Rheumatol*, 2003, 15(4), 469-75.

[2] Lourida, ES; Georgiadis, AN; Papavasiliou, EC; Papathanasiou, AI; Drosos, AA; Tselepis, AD. Patients with early rheumatoid arthritis exhibit elevated autoantibody titers against mildly oxidized low-density lipoprotein and exhibit decreased activity of the lipoprotein-associated phospholipase A2. *Arthritis Res. Ther.*, 2007, 9(1), R19.

[3] Gabriel, SE; Crowson, CS; Kremers, HM; Doran, MF; Turesson, C; O'Fallon, WM; Matteson, EL. Survival in rheumatoid arthritis: a population-based analysis of trends over 40 years. *Arthritis Rheum*, 2003, 48, 54-8.

[4] Symmons, DP. Looking back: rheumatoid arthritis - aetiology, occurrence and mortality. *Rheumatology*, 2005, 44, iv14-7.

[5] Goodson, N. Coronary artery disease and rheumatoid arthritis. Curr. Opin. *Rheumatol*, 2002, 14, 115-20.

[6] Van Doornum, S; McColl, G; Wicks, I. Accelerated atherosclerosis: an extraarticular feature of rheumatoid arthritis? *Arthritis Rheum*, 2002, 46, 862-73.

[7] Ritchlin, C. Psoriatic disease--from skin to bone. Nat. Clin. Pract. *Rheumatol*, 2007, 3, 698-706.

[8] Gonzalez-Juanatey, C; Llorca, J; Miranda-Filloy, JA; Amigo-Diaz, E; Testa, A; Garcia-Porrua, C; Martin, J; Gonzalez-Gay, MA. Endothelial dysfunction in psoriatic arthritis patients without clinically evident cardiovascular disease or classic atherosclerosis risk factors. *Arthritis Rheum.*, 2007, 57, 287-93.

[9] Kimhi, O; Caspi, D; Bornstein, NM; Maharshak, N; Gur, A; Arbel, Y; Comaneshter, D; Paran, D; Wigler, I; Levartovsky, D; Berliner, S; Elkayam, O. Prevalence and risk factors of atherosclerosis in patients with psoriatic arthritis. Semin. *Arthritis Rheum*, 2007, 36(4), 203-9.

[10] Hahn, BH; Grossman, J; Chen, W; McMahon, M. The pathogenesis of atherosclerosis in autoimmune rheumatic diseases: roles of inflammation and dyslipidemia. *J. Autoimmun*, 2007, 28, 69-75.

[11] Gállego, J; Martínez Vila, E; Muñoz, R. Patients at high risk for ischemic stroke: identification and actions. *Cerebrovasc. Dis.*, 2007, 24 Suppl 1, 49-63.

[12] Pearson, TA. New tools for coronary risk assessment: what are their advantages and limitations? *Circulation*, 2002, 105, 886-92.

[13] Steiner, G. Atherosclerosis in type 2 diabetes: a role for fibrate therapy? Diab. *Vasc. Dis. Res.*, 2007, 4, 368-74.

[14] Juonala, M; Viikari, JS; Rönnemaa, T; Marniemi, J; Jula, A; Loo, BM; Raitakari, OT. Associations of Dyslipidemias From Childhood to Adulthood With Carotid Intima-Media Thickness, Elasticity, and Brachial Flow-Mediated Dilatation in Adulthood. The Cardiovascular Risk in Young Finns Study. Arterioscler. *Thromb Vasc. Biol.*, 2008 Feb 28, [Epub ahead of print].

[15] Michos, ED; Vaidya, D; Gapstur, SM; Schreiner, PJ; Golden, SH; Wong, ND; Criqui, MH; Ouyang, P. Sex hormones, sex hormone binding globulin, and abdominal aortic calcification in women and men in the multi-ethnic study of atherosclerosis (MESA). *Atherosclerosis*, 2008, Feb 7, [Epub ahead of print].

[16] Assayag, EB; Bova, I; Kesler, A; Berliner, S; Shapira, I; Bornstein, NM. Erythrocyte aggregation as an early biomarker in patients with asymptomatic carotid stenosis. *Dis. Markers.*, 2008, 24, 33-9.

[17] de, Ferranti, SD; Rifai, N. C-reactive protein: a nontraditional serum marker of cardiovascular risk. Cardiovasc. *Pathol*, 2007, 16(1), 14-21.

[18] Kabuyama, Y; Kitamura, T; Yamaki, J; Homma, MK; Kikuchi, S; Homma, Y. Involvement of thioredoxin reductase 1 in the regulation of redox balance and viability of rheumatoid synovial cells. Biochem. Biophys. *Res. Commun.*, 2008, 367, 491-6.

[19] Firuzi, O; Fuksa, L; Spadaro, C; Bousová, I; Riccieri, V; Spadaro, A; Petrucci, R; Marrosu, G; Saso, L. Oxidative stress parameters in different systemic rheumatic diseases. *J. Pharm. Pharmacol.*, 2006, 58, 951-7.

[20] Spinetti, G; Kraenkel, N; Emanueli, C; Madeddu, P. Diabetes and Vessel Wall Remodeling: from Mechanistic Insights to Regenerative Therapies. *Cardiovasc. Res.*, 2008 Feb 15, [Epub ahead of print].

[21] Gracia-Sancho, J; Laviña, B; Rodríguez-Vilarrupla, A; García-Calderó, H; Fernández, M; Bosch, J; García-Pagán, JC. Increased oxidative stress in cirrhotic rat livers: A potential mechanism contributing to reduced nitric oxide bioavailability. *Hepatology*, 2007, Dec 10, [Epub ahead of print].

[22] Arnett, FC; Edworthy, SM; Bloch, DA; McShane, DJ; Fries, JF; Cooper, NS; Healey, LA; Kaplan, SR; Liang, MH; Luthra, HS; et al. The American Rheumatism Association 1987 revised criteria fort the classification of rheumatoid arthritis. *Arthritis Rheum*, 1988, 31, 315-24.

[23] Taylor, W; Gladman, D; Helliwell, Ph; Marchesoni, A; Mease Ph, Mielants, H. the CASPAR Study Group. Classification criteria for psoriatic arthritis. Development of new criteria from a large international study. *Arthritis Rheum.*, 2006, 54, 2665-73.

[24] Ryoo, S; Lemmon, CA; Soucy, KG; Gupta, G; White, AR; Nyhan, D; Shoukas, A; Romer, LH; Berkowitz, DE. Oxidized low-density lipoprotein-dependent endothelial arginase II activation contributes to impaired nitric oxide signaling. *Circ. Res.*, 2006, 99, 951-60.

[25] Flam, BR; Eichler, DC; Solomonson, LP. Endothelial nitric oxide production is tightly coupled to the citrulline-NO cycle. *Nitric. Oxide*, 2007, 17, 115-21.

[26] Durante, W; Johnson, FK; Johnson, RA. Arginase: a critical regulator of nitric oxide synthesis and vascular function. Clin. Exp. *Pharmacol, Physiol*, 2007, 34, 906-11.

[27] Ryoo, S; Gupta, G; Benjo, A; Lim, HK; Camara, A; Sikka, G; Lim, HK; Sohi, J; Santhanam, L; Soucy, K; Tuday, E; Baraban, E; Ilies, M; Gerstenblith, G; Nyhan, D; Shoukas, A; Christianson, DW; Alp, NJ; Champion, HC; Huso, D; Berkowitz, DE. Endothelial Arginase II. A Novel Target for the Treatment of Atherosclerosis. *Circ. Res.*, 2008, Feb 28, [Epub ahead of print]

[28] Nash, DT. Use of vascular ultrasound in clinical trials to evaluate new cardiovascular therapies. *J. Natl. Med. Assoc*, 2008, 100, 222-9.

[29] Agerholm-Larsen, B; Tybjaerg-Hansen, A; Schnohr, P; Steffensen, R; Nordestgaard, BG. Common cholesteryl ester transfer protein mutations, decreased HDL cholesterol, and possible decreased risk of ischemic heart disease: The Copenhagen City Heart Study. *Circulation*, 2000, 102, 2197-203.

Index

B

C

D

E

F

G

H

I

J

K

L

M

N

O

P

Q

R

S

T